Leisure Competence Measure: Adult Version
Professional Manual and Users' Guide

An Introduction to Measuring Outcomes in Therapeutic Recreation

Marita Kloseck, M.Sc., CTRS
Richard G. Crilly, M.D.

ISBN 0-9683306-0-6

Preface

This is a very challenging, yet exciting time for the therapeutic recreation profession. In many health care systems around the world increasing demand for accountability, a growing emphasis on evidence-based practice, and in some cases declining funding, require all health care professionals, including therapeutic recreation specialists, to provide much greater accountability for the services they deliver. As a result, the collection of outcome data that demonstrates the effectiveness, efficiency and quality of therapeutic recreation intervention is no longer optional. Measuring outcomes has become a necessity. Further, there has recently been a paradigm shift in health care, resulting in the implementation of new models of care, significant changes in professional practice and major changes in care delivery. Most notable is the increasing emphasis on client-centred care practices. Therefore, every therapeutic recreation practitioner must now become responsible for routinely incorporating the measurement of outcomes, as well as client and family satisfaction, into their daily practice.

The need for standardization and uniformity in assessment procedures and the delivery of therapeutic recreation intervention have also been recognized. The field, however, is still struggling with which outcomes to measure, how to measure them and how to interpret and utilize the findings. The Leisure Competence Measure (LCM) and this manual will afford therapeutic recreation professionals an objective way of documenting current levels of leisure functioning and demonstrating change over time. The LCM also provides the therapeutic recreation profession with a core set of leisure functioning measures, standardized definitions of terms and data that all therapeutic recreation professionals can then use in a similar way. This will allow more accurate comparison of therapeutic recreation intervention and program results among similar facilities and client groups.

While this is a challenging time for the profession, it is a great opportunity for therapeutic recreation professionals to guide the way in measuring psychosocial outcomes, an area identified by the American Congress of Rehabilitation Medicine and the American Academy of Physical Medicine and Rehabilitation as particularly lacking in well developed and rigorously tested measures. With the increased emphasis in health care today on social intervention, life satisfaction and community integration, an opening exists for the therapeutic recreation profession to position itself as a leader in advancing the measurement of psychosocial outcomes.

Marita Kloseck
Richard G. Crilly

Acknowledgements

Appreciation and thanks are extended to the many individuals involved in the development of the Leisure Competence Measure (LCM) and the production of this document. Elsa Lammers, Co-leader of the Essex, Kent & Lambton Inpatient/Outpatient Programs, London and St. Thomas Psychiatric Hospitals co-authored the LCM and was instrumental in the initial conceptualization, implementation and advancement of the LCM. Michael Kloseck, developer of software systems for a leading marketing firm in Vancouver, British Columbia collaborated with Dr. Gary Ellis, Dean, Department of Recreation and Leisure at the University of Utah, and developed the LCM software. Sheryl Dedman, Therapeutic Recreation Specialist at the Rotary Centre in Waterloo, Ontario was instrumental in beginning development of the paediatric version of the LCM. Linda Hutchinson-Troyer, Patient Therapy Co-ordinator for the Brain Injury Unit and Outpatient Therapy Services at the Kernan Hospital in Baltimore, Maryland initiated and refined the use of LCM indicators for goal achievement analysis and quality improvement purposes. Kerry Hofstede, Therapeutic Recreation Specialist on the Brain Injury Unit and Maureen Dow, Therapeutic Recreation Specialist in the Geriatric Day Hospital at Parkwood Hospital in London, Ontario were very enthusiastic about the potential of the LCM and extremely committed to ongoing validation and clinical application of the LCM. Elizabeth Davison, CTRS, West Park Hospital, Toronto, Ontario was most supportive of, and extensively involved in, LCM related research with a geriatric population. Dr. Jerry Jordan, Chair of the Department of Leisure Studies at Oklahoma State University and Dr. Jean Keller, Dean, College of Education at the University of North Texas shared their professional expertise, dedication and commitment without hesitation during the past eight years and caused this project to grow. Dr. Paul Stolee, Manager, Program Research and Evaluation, Regional Geriatric Program of South Western Ontario provided expertise on goal attainment scaling and use of this method in daily practice.

The Parkwood Hospital Foundation and the Ontario Ministry of Tourism and Recreation provided financial support that allowed extensive validation and refinement of the LCM. Credit must also be given to the many individuals and agencies who believed in the potential of the LCM and who were committed enough to share their comments and experiences regarding use of the LCM with their particular populations.

The LCM data system is still undergoing refinement. Your comments and suggestions are welcome.

A special thanks goes to Elsa Lammers for her insightful and very valuable editorial comments in preparing this manual for publication.

About the Authors . . . . .

Marita Kloseck, M.Sc., CTRS

Marita is completing her joint Ph.D. in Health Studies and Recreation/Leisure Studies at the University of Waterloo, Ontario, Canada. Her areas of specialization are health program evaluation, social psychology of leisure and therapeutic recreation. Marita has 17 years combined experience as a practitioner, consultant and researcher in the field of therapeutic recreation. She is a widely known consultant and trainer in outcome measurement related to therapeutic recreation in Canada and the United States and has been extremely instrumental in promoting accountability for therapeutic recreation specialists. Marita has won numerous national and international awards including a National Health Research and Development award from Health Canada, awards from the Ontario Recreation Society, the American Therapeutic Recreation Association, the National Recreation and Park Association in the United States and the World Leisure and Recreation Association. Marita is also actively involved in community development and mobilization initiatives around health issues. She is currently responsible for the development, implementation and evaluation of a new and innovative community-driven, integrated model of health service delivery for seniors.

Richard G. Crilly, M.D.

Dr. Richard Crilly did his medical and research training in the United Kingdom before moving to Canada in 1981. He is Associate Professor in the Division of Geriatric Medicine at the University of Western Ontario, Ontario, Canada. His interests range from osteoporosis to geriatric community program development. Dr. Crilly has extensive experience in geriatric rehabilitation, both in in-patient and geriatric day hospital settings. Until recently he was Director of the Regional Geriatric Program of South Western Ontario where his main interest was the development of community independence in geriatric assessment and management, and program evaluation. He has co-authored a number of chapters on osteoporosis in a variety of books, and has also published extensively in the areas of osteoporosis, the effect of exercise on function in the elderly and life satisfaction in the elderly. He also has a long-standing interest in the measurement of outcomes in geriatric rehabilitation programs. Dr. Crilly is currently involved in exploring ways in which evidence is, or is not, incorporated into clinical program delivery systems and is attempting to make geriatric programs more evidence-based.

What is the Leisure Competence Measure (LCM)?

The LCM is a standardized instrument designed to measure outcomes related to therapeutic recreation. The LCM has been conceptualized according to:

- ❑ rehabilitation theory operationalized through the International Classification of Impairment, Disability and Handicap (ICIDH) developed by the World Health Organization (WHO) in 1980
- ❑ the leisure-based philosophy for therapeutic recreation practice operationalized through the Leisure Ability Model
- ❑ the behavioural construct of competence

The LCM is intended to complement other therapeutic recreation tools and to categorize and summarize information gained through the initial therapeutic recreation assessment process.

The LCM:

* objectively measures client ability related to leisure functioning
* objectively captures change in client functioning over time
* guides therapeutic recreation intervention
* guides goal setting
* is consistent with the Functional Independence Measure (FIM)
* provides a basis for program evaluation
* assists in targeting the effective use of resources
* is simple to use with minimal time required!

The LCM assesses:

* leisure awareness
* leisure attitude
* leisure skills
* cultural/social behaviours
* interpersonal skills
* community integration skills
* social contact
* community participation

When fully developed, the LCM data system will consist of:

1. Leisure Competence Measure (paper pencil version; windows-based software)
2. Program evaluation/goal achievement components (through use of LCM indicators)
3. Computerized data base (providing regional, national and international comparative data on therapeutic recreation outcomes)

The LCM has been evaluated for:

* validity
* reliability
* feasibility
* sensitivity to change

What will the LCM do for you?

The LCM will:

- ☺ provide you with a standardized tool to measure outcomes related to therapeutic recreation
- ☺ provide you with an objective way to evaluate changes over time in client functioning
- ☺ allow you to compare the outcomes of your clients with many similar clients across a variety of settings
- ☺ help you to ensure compliance with standards established by accrediting bodies such as the Commission on Accreditation of Rehabilitation Facilities (CARF), the Joint Commission on Accreditation of Healthcare Organizations (JCAHO) and the Canadian Council on Health Services Accreditation (CCHSA)
- ☺ in it's consistency with the FIM, provide you with a recognized and accepted means of reporting at inter-disciplinary team rounds
- ☺ help guide therapeutic recreation intervention and help you to provide quality service to your clients
- ☺ provide you with a mechanism for program evaluation and a tool for continuous quality improvement
- ☺ help you make evidence-based decisions related to therapeutic recreation practice
- ☺ provide you with a simple to use, easy to learn and time effective tool for measuring outcomes, that can easily be incorporated into your daily practice
- ☺ provide accountability data to your team, administrators and funders

What will the LCM do for our profession?

The LCM will provide our profession with:

* a core set of leisure functioning measures, consistent definitions and information related to leisure functioning that all professionals interpret in a similar way
* a more accurate way of comparing TR intervention and program results among similar facilities and client populations
* a means of establishing a scientific basis for our profession
* one means of demonstrating the value of our contribution in what has become the era of evidence

The LCM computerized data base will:

* provide regional, national and international comparative data
* provide an international research base for therapeutic recreation

The LCM:

* has been rigorously tested, over time and demonstrates evidence of good validity, reliability, feasibility and sensitivity to change
* is simple to use, easily built into daily TR practice and useful across a variety of disabilities and settings

What professionals have to say about the LCM . . . . .

". . . . use of the LCM provides an excellent opportunity for recreation therapists to monitor outcomes achieved by their patients. This tool has the potential to provide recreation therapists with a comparative data base on a national level. It is a tool that you can utilize as part of your performance improvement and program evaluation reports for both CARF and JCAHO standards."

Linda Hutchinson-Troyer, MGA, CTRS
Patient Therapy Co-ordinator
Brain Injury and Outpatient Therapy Services
Kernan Hospital, Baltimore, Maryland U.S.A.

". . . . . in 1993, San Diego Rehabilitation Institute (SDRI) incorporated the LCM as part of our Therapeutic Recreation Department's assessment and documentation system. As San Diego became one of the more highly competitive managed markets, consumers were demanding proof of outcomes. In 1994, our clinical services team members were challenged by our medical staff to enlarge our outcome areas to include areas such as life satisfaction, health, leisure and psychosocial, with hopes that this would enable our hospital to demonstrate the extra services provided at SDRI. The LCM, we were already using, was found to be the most comprehensive outcome tool so we chose to continue with that scale. We have utilized the LCM mostly in our assessment and documentation system, however, I see great potential for the LCM in the areas of program evaluation, and for valuable research in the field of therapeutic recreation.

Mary Williams, CTRS, RTC
Director, Therapeutic Recreation
San Diego Rehabilitation Institute
San Diego, California, U.S.A.

". . . . . Leisure is an experience that can occur at any time, not necessarily obtained through participation in any particular activity. One's ability to experience "true" leisure is drastically impacted by traumatic brain injury. Therapeutic recreation specialists recognize the need to facilitate the restoration of the physical, cognitive, emotional and social skills required. However, until recently many professionals have not accepted the need to measure clients' progress. The LCM is an innovative measurement system that provides TRSs with the opportunity to determine admission and discharge scores, as well as change over time. A great way to demonstrate outcomes!"

Kerry Hofstede, Hons. B.A.
Therapeutic Recreation Specialist
Brain Injury Program, Parkwood Hospital
London, Ontario, Canada

". . . . . a tool (LCM) that directly impacts service!"

Workshop Participant
Documenting Outcomes in Therapeutic Recreation Workshop
COLUMBIA Spalding Rehabilitation Hospital System
Colorado, U.S.A.

". . . . .the LCM provides a comprehensive overview of the social and leisure-related needs that must be addressed in a client's care plan. When used in long-term care, the LCM can be helpful in ensuring that all clients receive the type of treatment and care that they require - be it rehabilitative, educational, diversionary or life-enriching sensory stimulation."

Nathalie Guerin, M.A.
Activity Assistant
Bethania Mennonite Personal Care Home
Winnipeg, Manitoba, Canada

". . . . . the LCM is an excellent assessment tool that measures more than just activity. It focuses on all of the behaviours clients must possess to be successful in their leisure. By measuring initially, and over time, clinicians are able to demonstrate change and outcomes in client functioning that lead to successful leisure involvement."

Elizabeth Davison, M.A., CTRS
West Park Hospital
Toronto, Ontario, Canada

". . . . . the LCM is great! Other clinicians in rehabilitation settings find it easy to understand due to its similar format to the F.I.M. - and it's a Canadian tool!"

Jennifer Ertel, Recreation Therapist
G.F. Strong Centre
Vancouver, British Columbia, Canada

". . . . . the LCM was one of the first tools which truly provided a link for the CTRS within the physical rehabilitation professional circle. Its compatible UDS/FIM style ratings have given much credibility to our discipline as we constantly strive to provide the same functional outcomes as our rehabilitation teammates."

Cheryl Frazier, CTRS
Director of Clinical Services
St. Vincent/North Rehabilitation Hospital
Sherwood, Arkansas, U.S.A.

". . . . . the LCM is a helpful and valuable instrument that guides client-centred intervention by drawing on the professional knowledge and clinical expertise of therapeutic recreation practitioners, focuses on the abilities, needs and interests of our clients and monitors the achievement of client goals and progress over time."

Paula Cassin, Manager
Community Outreach Support Service
Brain Injury Community Re-Entry (Niagara) Inc.
St. Catharines, Ontario, Canada

". . . . . health facilities are putting increasing demands on therapeutic recreation practitioners to be accountable and document change over time. The LCM provides TR practitioners with a valuable tool that can be used to measure outcomes with adolescents with disabilities. However, there continues to be a lack of tools designed and tested to measure outcomes in the younger paediatric population. Hopefully the paediatric version of the LCM, currently under development, will fill this gap."

Sheryl Dedman, B.Sc.
Therapeutic Recreation Specialist
The Rotary Childrens' Centre
Waterloo, Ontario, Canada

". . . . . the LCM has promoted greater consistency and continuity in all recreation therapists' discussions at client case conferences. We now all speak the same language related to leisure issues. Other care team members have a greater understanding of leisure and the benefits of meaningful leisure experiences."

Val Bakowski, D.Sc., B.A., ACC
Director of Therapeutic Recreation
Bethania Mennonite Personal Care Home/
Concordia Hospital
Winnipeg, Manitoba, Canada

". . . . . our department has been using the LCM for 4 and a half years. Not only has the LCM helped us with documentation, but this tool has given us the measurable outcomes that are now required for all health professionals. The LCM's consistency with the FIM gives us professional credibility and puts us on the same level with other inter-disciplinary team members. They understand the "language" and better understand the contribution our profession has to make. The LCM is also helpful for our quarterly quality assurance reporting."

Debbie Cummings, CTRS
Department Head, Therapeutic Recreation
St. Vincent/North Rehabilitation Hospital
Sherwood, Arkansas, U.S.A.

Common Myths

1. *My day is usually very busy, from the moment I arrive at work in the morning. I don't have the time to spend on documentation. Besides, it is much more important for me to spend direct time with my clients, than to spend time away from my clients doing paperwork.*

   False. It is critically important for all therapeutic recreation practitioners to conduct comprehensive assessments and document functional and behavioural change, over time, of their clients. This information is necessary for ensuring a quality therapeutic recreation service, consumer protection, legal accountability, as well as to provide accountability to funders, accrediting bodies and one's own agency. If you want to keep your job, it is absolutely necessary to have good documentation!

2. *I work in a long-term care facility. Our goals are not rehabilitative like those in more acute, clinical settings, so there isn't the same need to document client progress.*

   False. All therapeutic recreation practitioners, no matter what their setting or population, have a responsibility to provide accurate, timely and regular documentation on each of their clients. Whether TRSs are working toward improving (rehabilitation), maintaining (long-term care), or minimizing a decrease in (Alzheimer units; special care units) physical, cognitive and/or social functioning of their clients, this documentation helps to ensure that programs and intervention provided are suited to client abilities, needs and interests.

Common Myths

3. *My clients are here such a short time and the turnover of clients is so high and so quick that I can barely keep up with my assessments. I don't have time to set goals with my clients.*

False. It is still important to set *reasonable* goals for your clients (otherwise why are we working here in the first place), taking into consideration of course, such factors as your setting, length of stay, prognosis of the client, discharge plans, etc. Most short-stay units are part of a larger system or continuum of care and often clients are transferred from one facility to another. The information you collect will be most helpful (and appreciated) by the next therapeutic recreation specialist who might be working with the same client. Collecting and forwarding this information also benefits the client, in that they are not subjected to having to go through the entire assessment process again.

Common Myths

4. *My clients can, and should make their own choices. All I have to do is observe them and work with them to help them join in community activities. This is a better way to empower individuals and a better way to spend my time; all that extra paperwork is really not necessary.*

False. Although we believe strongly in client empowerment, many of the individuals in rehabilitation, long-term care, psychiatric and community settings are not yet at this stage. Much work needs to be done to work collaboratively with these individuals to build their abilities, and to modify or develop new interests before independent and self-sustaining leisure involvement can be expected. For some clients, this might never happen, but they still have needs that we must strive to meet. It is important to(1) objectively identify and document what abilities our clients have when we begin to work with them, (2) together with our clients determine what we are working toward, and (3) collaboratively monitor what progress the client is making toward achieving the goals they have set for themselves. It is the responsibility of the therapeutic recreation specialist to ensure that client abilities are matched with client interests to ensure a successful leisure experience, rather than taking a "hit and miss" (let's see what happens as we go along) approach that may well negatively impact the client.

Table of Contents

Leisure Competence Measure: Professional Manual and Users' Guide

Page

List of Tables

List of Figures

Page

About this Manual . . . .

We originally intended this as simply a guide to the use of the LCM. However, experience in training sessions and many discussions with therapeutic recreation practitioners in the field, has underlined the need for some guidance in several areas of importance to our profession. Many practitioners have asked about accountability, how can outcomes be measured, what kind of documentation is required and how can we demonstrate the value of our role as a core service. In response we have introduced into this manual some discussion on these topics. Our idea was to introduce practitioners to some concepts that they might not be familiar with, and to provide a conceptual framework for thought and action to give insight into the overall process of therapeutic recreation intervention. We are not able, in a manual such as this, to go into depth, but hope that what we provide will help practitioners identify for themselves areas of interest and areas where they would like to learn more. There are many excellent references available on each of these topics. To encourage practitioners, and help identify available resources, we provide relevant references for most of these topics.

Chapters 1 and 2 of this manual provide more general conceptual and theoretical information. Chapters 3, 4 and 5 are specific to the LCM and provide numerous actual case examples to help therapeutic recreation practitioners learn how to administer, score and interpret the LCM, as well as set goals and objectively document the achievement of goals.

The LCM is still undergoing refinement and we welcome any suggestions that you may have.

CHAPTER 1
Introduction to Measuring Outcomes

SUMMARY

- *A growing demand for accountability and evidence-based decision making has put increasing pressure on health care systems to re-evaluate the essential components of care.*
- *Health professionals are now required to provide outcome data that demonstrate the effectiveness, efficiency and quality of their services.*
- *Uniformity and standardization are necessary in the profession's approach to assessment and outcome measurement in order to accurately compare different therapeutic recreation interventions and programs.*
- *Instruments selected and utilized for assessment and outcome measurement purposes should provide evidence of rigorous testing, including detailed information on the instruments' validity, reliability, feasibility and sensitivity results.*
- *Goal setting, based on an assessment of a client's general functioning, leisure functioning and personal interests, is central to both the planning of therapeutic intervention and program evaluation.*
- *Therapeutic recreation practitioners must take responsibility for, and make a commitment to, ensuring that change in leisure functioning of their clients is objectively measured and routinely incorporated into their daily therapeutic recreation practice.*

Chapter 1
Introduction to Measuring Outcomes

Introduction

During the past decade, with the broadening definition of health and expansion of health-related services, there has been a shift toward including psychosocial outcomes in medical evaluation systems within institutions, as part of community-based services and as part of community mobilization efforts. In the past, medical concerns, physical function and activities of daily living (adls) were considered of primary concern.. More recently, the importance of an individual with a disability acquiring the necessary knowledge, skills and abilities to participate fully in society following intervention or completion of a rehabilitation program has been recognized.[1,2,3,4,5,6,7] Similarly, health-related research is now focusing on the wider issues of socialization, life satisfaction and quality of life of individuals with disabilities. In addition, greater emphasis is being placed on long-term follow-up of individuals discharged from health programs and facilities. This is particularly true for the elderly who are more frequent users of social support services, and who are at greater risk for chronic disease than the general population.[8,9]

Consistent with this change in focus, recent funding realities have begun to put pressure on current health care systems in Canada and the United States to re-evaluate the essential components of care that are necessary to ensure the greatest success in health programs and to ensure optimal functioning of individuals with disabilities. As a result, allied health professionals are increasingly called upon to provide outcome data that demonstrates the effectiveness, efficiency and quality of their services.[3,10,11] This, in turn raises new conceptual and outcome measurement issues in the delivery of health-related services.

Forer[12] argues that in order to justify, maintain or expand funding it is essential "to describe the functional level of clients upon entry into the program, the amount of functional gain made within the program, as well as after discharge, and the final functional level attained by clients at follow-up" (p. 123). Of primary interest to funding sources is the effectiveness of programs in minimizing long-term medical and social support costs by enabling individuals with disabilities to live independently, with the least amount of assistance or supervision, following completion of health-related programs.[13] In order to accurately document functional gains achieved by individuals, improved instruments and evaluation procedures are necessary to measure concepts such as community integration, social adjustment, life satisfaction and quality of life following intervention and treatment programs.[4,11,14,15]

Therapeutic recreation professionals must be responsive to these identified needs and build into their daily clinical practice and service delivery systems an objective means of capturing the leisure functioning status of the individuals with whom they work. This will allow evaluation of changes in leisure functioning that may result from therapeutic recreation intervention or treatment. Not only is this required to ensure compliance with the Commission on Accreditation of Rehabilitation Facilities (CARF), the Joint Commission on Accreditation of Healthcare Organizations (JCAHO) and the Canadian Council on Health Services Accreditation (CCHSA) standards, but also to provide consumers with a quality service that meets their unique needs, as well as support therapeutic recreation as an essential professional service. In the process of measuring outcomes, care must be taken to ensure that psychometrically sound instruments are utilized, standards consistent with the requirements of CARF, JCAHO, CCHSA and other accrediting bodies are followed, and that only evidence-based information is utilized to make decisions related to therapeutic recreation practice.

The Need for Standardization

In order to determine the effectiveness and efficiency of therapeutic recreation interventions it is necessary to measure change over time in a standardized fashion to ascertain what works and what doesn't for clients with particular diagnoses and problems. Similarly, when comparing programs, standardization of measurements is necessary to allow valid comparisons to be made. To ensure that inferences made from these comparisons are accurate, it is important that the same outcomes are measured, that outcomes are measured in a consistent fashion, and that results are interpreted in similar ways.

Among the challenges currently facing the therapeutic recreation profession are the absence of uniformity and standardization in assessment procedures, the absence of uniformity in the delivery of therapeutic recreation intervention, and the lack of a consistent approach to measuring outcomes and program effectiveness. The profession is continuing to struggle with, and has not yet reached agreement on: (1) which core domains of functioning to assess; (2) a standardized approach to use to assess client abilities, needs and interests; (3) which instruments or tools to use to assess functioning in specific domains; (4) the type, duration and frequency of intervention necessary to ensure optimal leisure functioning of individuals with various disabilities; and (5) how to measure change over time. As a result, many therapeutic recreation practitioners are responding to their facilities' requirement for increased accountability by developing their own assessment tools and protocols for service delivery. This lack of uniformity within the profession and the resulting inconsistencies in domains being measured, inconsistencies in definitions of terms, and use of inadequately tested measures make it impossible to evaluate the changes that may result from therapeutic recreation intervention. This renders information from shared data bases meaningless and severely hinders the profession's ability to demonstrate the efficacy of therapeutic recreation.

Fuhrer[3] argues that "in the literature of evaluation research outcomes are understood to result from defined intervention" (p. 1) and although improvements are often observed following rehabilitation, improvements become outcomes "only if we infer that the changes resulted from the services provided" (p. 3). Necessary requisites, then, are to clearly define the specific type of intervention that should be provided, the specific type of outcomes expected from these interventions and standardized ways of measuring them.

Adding to the challenges of standardizing care delivery procedures within the profession, is the significant change that the health care system is currently undergoing in many countries (Figure 1). Changes in organizational structures of health care facilities, changes in professional practice and implementation of new models of care are forcing the profession to re-examine the services provided and to explore the "best fit" for the therapeutic recreation profession in the new health delivery systems being established. Recognizing the need for ongoing accountability, the profession must now determine, and reach agreement on, which components of the therapeutic recreation process are unique to the profession, which components of the therapeutic recreation process have the greatest impact on optimizing client leisure functioning, how to avoid duplication of services provided by other professional disciplines and how to best complement the services and care provided by other members of the interdisciplinary team.

Also important to consider is the shift toward more client-centred and client-driven practices by all professions. This requires therapeutic recreation practitioners not only to measure satisfaction levels of clients and their families in a consistent fashion, but also to ensure that clients and their families play an integral role in all phases of the therapeutic recreation process. Mechanisms must be developed which guarantee client and family inclusion in the assessment process, care planning, treatment and intervention phase, as well as program evaluation. Alternative models of client-focused, client-centred and client-driven approaches to service delivery are currently being examined by numerous health professions. Standardizing therapeutic recreation procedures and techniques is critical in order to strengthen the profession's scientifically established body of knowledge and, more importantly, to support the carrying out of efficacy research related to therapeutic recreation that is so desperately needed during this time of significant change and restructuring in health care (Figure 2). Interestingly, although the Leisure Competence Measure (LCM) was not designed to redefine leisure education techniques and practices but rather document client responses to existing leisure education approaches outlined in leisure literature[23,24,25] one of the requests received most often from practitioners using the LCM is for a manual outlining specific interventions designed to enhance client functioning in each of the eight domains represented by the LCM. Standardization of LCM materials, administration, scoring and interpretation of results, as well as standardizing therapeutic recreation intervention will make it possible to create large comparative data bases consisting

FIGURE 1. CURRENT TRENDS IN HEALTH CARE

Greater pressure on health systems to determine core components of care, that are necessary to optimize client functioning for specific programs

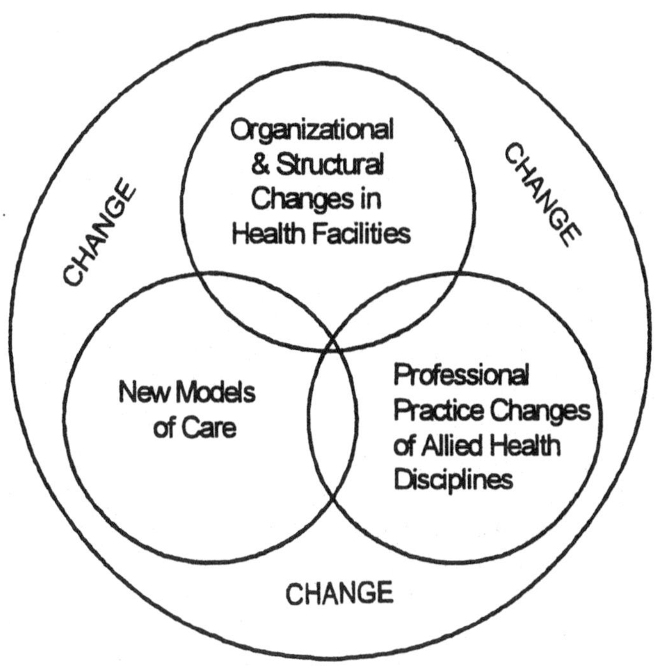

Greater pressure on allied health professionals to provide outcome data that demonstrates the effectiveness, efficiency and quality of their services, and justifies their inclusion as a core service

FIGURE 2. EVIDENCE-BASED ACCOUNTABILITY PARADIGM

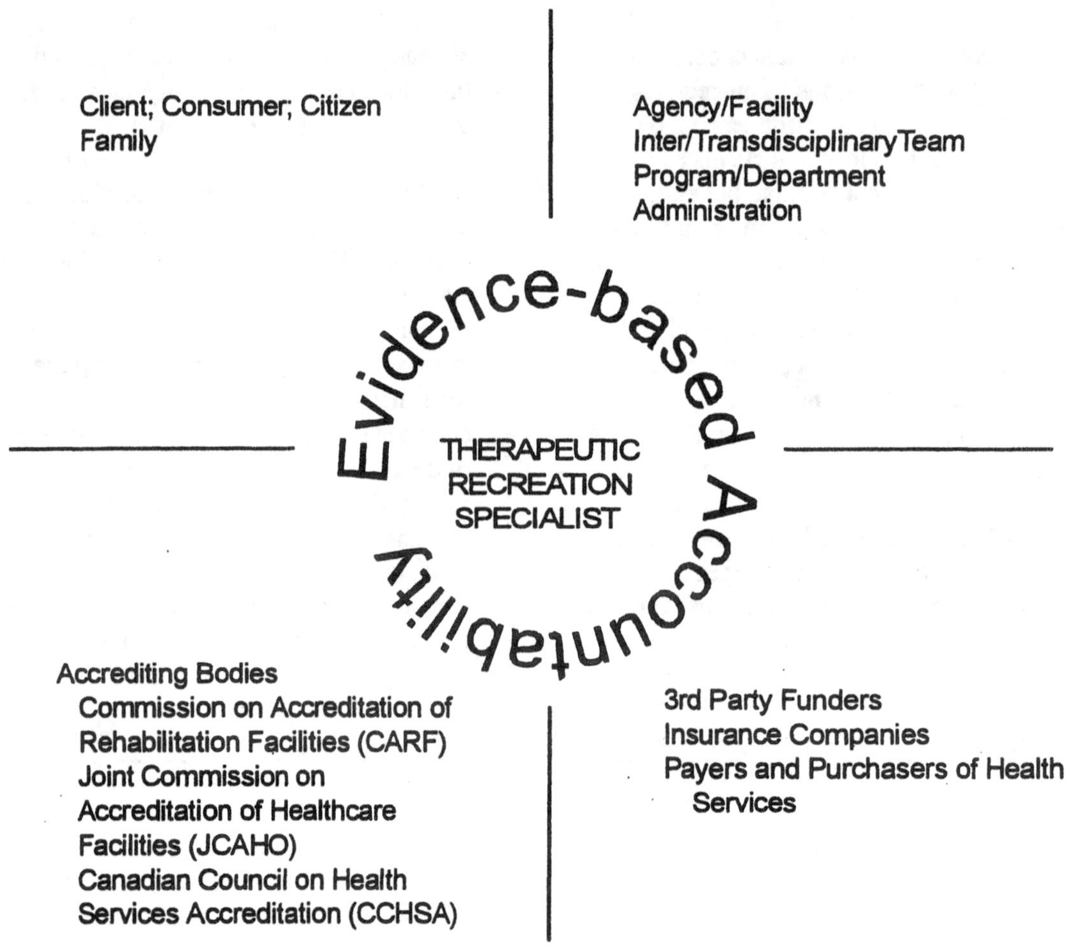

of many types of clients across a variety of settings. A tremendous need exists for standardized outcome measures in therapeutic recreation. The LCM provides practitioners with one means of quantifying leisure functioning, that is, representing specific client characteristics or attributes related to leisure functioning with numerical scores, and subsequently documenting change in functioning over time. The LCM, based on the results of testing completed to date, may be of use in measuring changes in leisure competence of clients in community-based or institutional settings[16,27] and represents a first step towards establishing a scientific base for our profession.

Psychometric and Measurement Considerations

One of the major criticisms found consistently throughout the medical and leisure literature is that few available psychosocial instruments have undergone the rigorous development and testing that is necessary to allow for accurate and dependable measurement of changes in the functional status of individuals.[3,4,16] In response to this identified need for improved health measures, the American Academy of Physical Medicine and Rehabilitation[4] developed interdisciplinary standards for instrument development in rehabilitation. These standards provide guidelines for, among other things, the development of instruments, reliability and validity testing, the development of accompanying manuals and the use of instruments by professionals. The LCM was developed according to these standards, as well as the standards for educational and psychological tests developed by the American Psychological Association.[17]

When selecting instruments for assessment purposes or for measuring outcomes, the selected instruments and their support material should provide evidence of rigorous testing and, at the very minimum, provide the validity and reliability evidence outlined in subsequent sections. The following sections were not intended to comprehensively discuss psychometric theory and principles, but rather to provide therapeutic recreation practitioners with a very brief introduction to the critical elements that must be considered when selecting instruments for use, modifying existing instruments for use, or developing one's own instrument. Without this basic and very important information, viable and dependable inferences regarding client functioning cannot be made. Excellent resources are available for readers wishing to read further on this topic. For those readers interested in more detailed information on psychometric theory and instrument development, additional resources related to this topic are referenced at the end of the chapter.

Validity

Validity is commonly defined as the extent to which an instrument accurately measures the domain (construct) which it is intended to measure.[18,19,20,21] It is important to note that instrument validation is a continuous process, carried out over time. New findings and conclusions from ongoing testing lend support (or lack of support) to existing evidence regarding the validity of inferences and conclusions that can be drawn from test scores. Instruments selected and utilized for assessment and outcome measurement purposes should have well documented validity. It is important to remember that an instrument is only valid for the particular population with which the instrument has been evaluated. The validation sample should match the client group for whom the instrument is intended to be used. Whether a new instrument is being developed for a specific purpose or an existing tool is chosen, comprehensive testing of various types of validity is required. Evidence of the following validity types should be available:

- ❑ Content Validity
- ❑ Criterion-Related Validity
  - Concurrent Validity
  - Predictive Validity
- ❑ Construct Validity
- ❑ Clinical or Prescriptive Validity

Each of these types of validity is outlined in more detail in Table 1. Validity testing of the LCM is described in Chapter 3. Results of ongoing testing conducted to date suggest that valid inferences regarding leisure competence may be made based on LCM scores.[16]

While content, criterion-related and construct validity are the more familiar forms of validity, references to clinical validity are more common in rehabilitation and evaluation literature. According to Johnston, Keith and Hinderer[4] and Silva[22] clinical or prescriptive validity is an often overlooked form of validity that should also be considered when developing instruments for use in clinical settings. This type of validity examines the extent to which

TABLE 1. TYPES OF VALIDITY

TYPE OF VALIDITY	DESCRIPTION	COMMENTS
CONTENT VALIDITY	This type of validity examines how adequately the instrument measures the attribute or behavioural domain of interest.	Support material should be provided for: ✔ how the items included in the instrument were chosen ✔ procedures that were followed to ensure that the instrument is appropriate and representative of the construct being measured
CRITERION-RELATED VALIDITY	There are 2 types of criterion-related validity: Concurrent Validity examines the degree to which scores obtained using a specific instrument correlate with some important criterion *occurring at the same time.* Predictive Validity examines the degree to which scores obtained using a specific instrument are *able to predict something of importance in the future.*	This type of validity examines how well the scores obtained by using the instrument correlate with or fail to correlate with those things one would expect them to correlate with. For example, do higher LCM scores correlate with cognitive status, higher life satisfaction scores and lower depression scores, etc. as one intuitively would expect them to?
CONSTRUCT VALIDITY	This type of validity examines how well scores obtained by using a specific instrument are consistent with underlying theories related to the instrument's content and construct of interest.	This is the most complex form of validity to establish. It is established over time by, among other things,: ✔ building a series of relationships ✔ differentiating the construct of interest from confounding variables (divergent/ discriminant validity) ✔ testing the instrument in a variety of settings and with a variety of populations so that generalizations can be made beyond a narrow scope, to the population in general, etc.
CLINICAL OR PRESCRIPTIVE VALIDITY	This type of validity examines how useful an instrument is for specific clinical purposes.	Use of the instrument should impact the planning of health-related programs and result in more effective intervention or treatment, as well as better client outcomes.

an instrument is "useful for specific clinical interventions for individuals. At a minimum clinical validity implies that use of a measure alters planning of rehabilitative treatments or support intervention"[4] (p. S-8). The LCM was designed to categorize and summarize baseline information related to leisure functioning of clients, guide intervention (based upon the results of initial LCM ratings), monitor client progress over time and assist therapeutic recreation professionals in modifying intervention to maximize independent leisure functioning. Formal testing of the clinical validity of the LCM is currently underway. Results of validity testing of the LCM, conducted to date, are outlined in Chapter 3.

Reliability

Reliability refers to measurement error and whether scores obtained by using an instrument, at different times and with different practitioners, are dependable, consistent and repeatable.[4,18,21,22] Instruments selected for use in therapeutic recreation practice should provide information regarding the following types of reliability:

- ❑ Test-Retest Reliability
- ❑ Alternative Forms or Parallel Forms Reliability
- ❑ Split-Half Reliability
- ❑ Inter-Item Consistency
- ❑ Inter-Rater Reliability

When selecting an instrument for clinical use, professionals should look for a high reliability coefficient. More detailed information regarding each of these types of reliability may be found in Table 2. Results of reliability testing conducted with the LCM are described in Chapter 3. Testing results to date support the LCM as an instrument that produces reliable and dependable scores.[16]

When selecting an instrument to meet their needs, professionals should look for the following information:

- ❑ a description of the diagnostic group with which the instrument was tested
- ❑ a description of the type of reliability being measured
- ❑ a description of the method that was used to determine reliability results
- ❑ a description of what exactly the instrument is intended to measure
- ❑ how to administer, score, and interpret the results obtained using the instrument
- ❑ any limitations or cautions outlined regarding use of the instrument

Testing reliability can be complex and is open to problems or "threats" to the validity of the conclusions drawn. For readers interested in more information on threats to validity, a number of excellent resources are available. Additional references are listed at the end of this chapter.

Feasibility

The feasibility of the instrument, that is, determining if using the instrument is possible, practical and worthwhile, is also an important consideration. Factors to consider include the time it takes to learn to utilize an instrument, the time it takes per client to complete the instrument, cost, etc. The LCM has been found to be feasible in various clinical settings, being easily incorporated into daily practice with minimum impact on time.

Sensitivity to Change

Sensitivity to change is a critical consideration in measures used to determine

TABLE 2. TYPES OF RELIABILITY

TYPE OF RELIABILITY	DESCRIPTION	COMMENTS
TEST-RETEST RELIABILITY	This type of reliability examines the consistency and dependability of an instrument. One instrument is administered on two separate occasions to the same client.	It is generally recommended that the time of the second administration not exceed 6 months. It is therefore important to look for information on administration times of the instrument. Good test-retest reliability indicates that very similar scores are obtained when the scale is administered twice on different occasions (providing there has been no intervention).
ALTERNATIVE OR PARALLEL FORMS RELIABILITY	With this type of reliability, two different versions or forms of an instrument measuring the same construct are administered to the same client.	This type of reliability is better than test-retest reliability because it decreases the possibility that memory will influence the answers and therefore produce a higher reliability estimate. However, the limitation is that often alternative forms are not available to measure the same construct.
SPLIT-HALF RELIABILITY	With this type of reliability one instrument is divided in two (usually by odd and even numbers) and one half of the instrument is administered at one point in time; the second half at a later point in time. Other ways of dividing an instrument include dividing it into first and second halves or randomly separating the items or questions into two groups.	Look for information on how the instrument was divided. This method and the above two methods (test-retest and alternative or parallel forms reliability) provide similar information.
INTER-ITEM CONSISTENCY	This type of reliability examines how well the individual items of an instrument reflect the common underlying construct that the instrument is trying to measure.	Inter-item consistency implies reasonable homogeneity in the construct being assessed.
INTER-RATER RELIABILITY	This type of reliability is used when the instrument is to be administered by an observer (vs. a self-report measure) and examines the degree to which scores obtained by one rater are consistent with scores obtained by another rater, for the same client.	Without a relatively high level of agreement among raters, it is difficult to make accurate statements about a client's behaviour. It is important to look for information on whether the ratings were done "blind" and when the ratings were made.

the effects of treatment. There are two criteria which need to be reconciled in the design of a tool. Firstly, the differences between different scores have to be great enough to have some real-life significance. Secondly, the differences need to be small enough for interventions to be realistically expected to produce a change. The LCM has been designed to satisfy these criteria. Although by using the LCM, change can be shown to occur during a rehabilitation program,[16,27] research is needed to make the central link between the therapeutic recreation intervention provided and the change that occurs.

Sensitivity to Diagnosis

The LCM is not a diagnostic tool. Nevertheless, being able to identify certain patterns of leisure dysfunction that are associated with specific diagnoses implies that the LCM is sensitive to the different needs of those with different problems thereby reinforcing the value of assessment and tailored therapeutic approaches. One size does not fit all, and simply identifying areas of interest without a full assessment of client abilities is inadequate. Intuitively, in the areas of traumatic brain injury, spinal cord injury and other specialized forms of rehabilitation, one would expect client abilities (cognitive and physical) and response to intervention to vary significantly depending upon a client's diagnosis. It is therefore important that the LCM is sensitive to picking up these differences. Preliminary studies designed to examine the sensitivity of the LCM[27] have demonstrated the LCM's ability to discriminate between diagnostic categories and disability levels.

Equal-Interval versus Approximately Equal-Interval Level Scales

Another area that requires brief mention is the use of equal interval versus approximately equal-interval level scales. Equal interval scales are like the measurement of distance, where each metre is the same. In the LCM however, being a descriptive scale, it is impossible to show that the distance from a score of 3 to a score of 4, for example, reflects precisely the same amount of change as moving from a score of 6 to 7. Such scales are at best, approximately equal interval scales.

While there is lack of consensus regarding the accuracy of estimating changes in approximately equal-interval level scales, this approach is considered defensible in the behavioural and social sciences. Johnston, Keith and Hinderer[4] argue that "larger samples, higher significance levels and special statistical models can be used to minimize the impact of imperfectly-equal intervals in gain scores" (p. S-19). The LCM is approximately equal-interval in that the representative behaviours of leisure competence that differentiate each of the seven levels of functioning (7=complete independence; 1=total dependence) are hierarchically ordered with each level being distinguished from the next by specific goals that must be achieved. Therefore, consistent with rehabilitation literature, the LCM is being treated as an interval level scale.

It is important for test users to understand the strengths and weaknesses of an instrument so they can evaluate the appropriateness of the instrument's use in various settings and for various purposes. More detailed information on the strengths and weaknesses of the LCM may be found in subsequent chapters.

Measuring Client Capabilities versus Actual Performance

A necessary consideration, according to rehabilitation, social gerontological and leisure literature is the importance of distinguishing between two types of approaches used in the measurement of outcomes; measurement of individual capabilities versus measurement of actual performance.[1, 16,28,29,30,31,32] On measures of capability, a rater documents the ability of the client to carry out a particular task in a specified environment. For example, the therapeutic recreation practitioner documents whether a client, while in a treatment setting, can independently or dependently demonstrate the required skills, knowledge and/or behaviours. General capability is inferred from specific examples of client performance, usually in simulated situations. Measurement of actual performance, on the other hand, documents not only change in functioning from admission to discharge but on follow-up provides evidence of the effectiveness, or lack of success of the intervention provided, in enabling one's client to live in the community independently.[32] Although this is a somewhat oversimplified definition (there are many factors in addition to treatment that may potentially influence actual performance), this type of measurement approach does provide the necessary foundation for examining a client's ability to live successfully in the community. The LCM is designed to measure leisure functioning in both real and simulated situations. The first five subscales (e.g., leisure awareness, leisure attitude, leisure skills, cultural/social behaviours, interpersonal skills) measure a client's capabilities or "readiness for" community re-entry or optimal performance in leisure. The sixth scale (community integration skills) examines the client's ability to translate the skills learned into a real-life setting. The remaining two subscales (social contact, community participation) measure actual levels of engagement in social and leisure opportunities, by the client. If the LCM is utilized post-discharge to obtain information on individual functioning once the client has returned home, the effectiveness and efficacy of therapeutic recreation intervention may be examined.

Wagner[32] argues that the capability approach, alone, "often gives a distorted view of the outcome picture" (p. 25). For example, a client who is capable of initiating, planning and following through with leisure activities while in a treatment setting, but who does not take part in activities once they are discharged home, continues to have difficulties with participation at the community level. Wagner[32] contends that measuring actual performance, whenever possible, is the preferred approach because it allows therapists to identify the problems remaining following the treatment process, so that the intervention can be modified to better address existing client needs.

In conclusion, we must say this section was by no means intended to provide in-depth information on psychometric and measurement considerations, but rather to simply highlight, for therapeutic recreation practitioners, some of the more critical factors that must be taken into account when selecting, modifying or developing instruments for professional purposes, or when attempting to measure outcomes related to leisure functioning achieved by their clients. Many excellent resources are available on each of these topics. Some of these references are provided at the end of this chapter.

Assessment versus Outcome Measurement

It is important to distinguish between the assessment process and measuring outcomes in therapeutic recreation. One approach provides baseline information regarding client functioning, the other examines the impact of specific treatment or intervention for the individual. Each of these approaches are discussed in more detail below and in subsequent sections of this manual

Assessment

Assessment provides baseline information regarding a client's general functioning (e.g., physical and cognitive functioning) as well as specific leisure functioning and individual preferences. This allows us to better identify specific strengths, as well as areas of concern, and to set measurable goals with our clients. Functional assessment in therapeutic recreation should focus on cognitive, affective and

FIGURE 3. ASSESSMENT CONSIDERATIONS IN THERAPEUTIC RECREATION

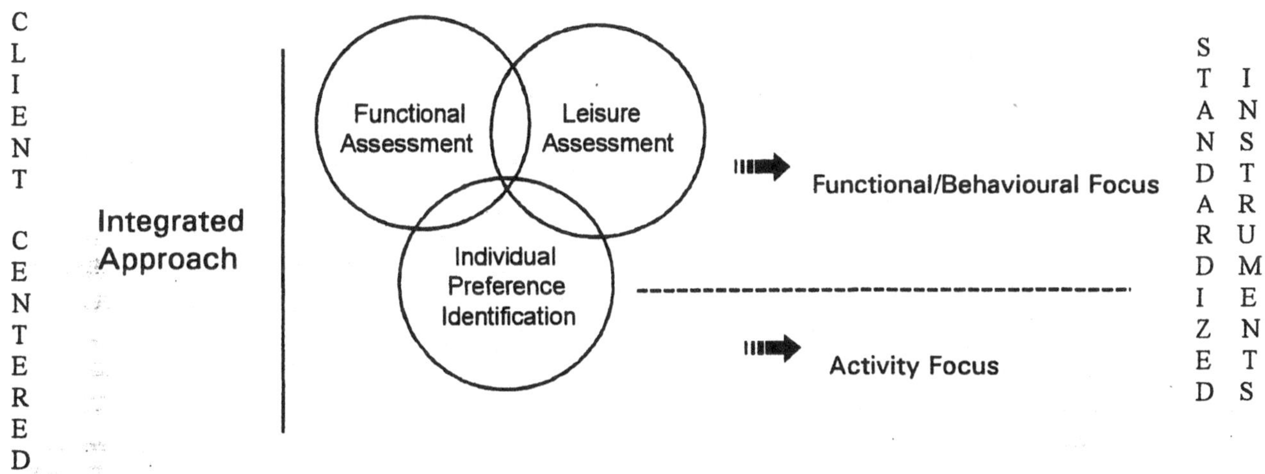

Note: Only by blending all three spheres into a truly integrated approach, can client-centred goal setting be accomplished. Concentrating solely on interests of clients (activity focus) regardless of ability is inadequate. There must be a close fit between a client's general functioning and leisure functioning capability, and a client's identified interests must be realistic in view of any limitation in leisure related capabilities.

TABLE 3. EXAMPLES OF NECESSARY FUNCTIONAL ANTECEDENTS TO SUCCESSFUL LEISURE INVOLVEMENT

Cognitive Domain	judgement; decision-making ability; attention span; short and long term memory; orientation; learning; ability to communicate thoughts, ideas and feelings; etc.
Affective Domain	ability to work co-operatively with others; group interaction skills; etc.
Psycho-motor Domain	fine/gross motor control; hand/eye co-ordination; hearing; vision; ambulation; balance; etc.

psycho-motor domains (Table 3). Functional ability is a necessary antecedent to leisure involvement and the attainment of a personally satisfying and meaningful lifestyle.

The leisure assessment is intended to gather information related to client leisure needs and abilities. The leisure assessment generally focuses on skills, knowledge and attitudes related to leisure and required to facilitate successful leisure participation and an independent lifestyle. It also provides a guide to leisure education, activity modification needs, identification of barriers to participation and assists in facilitating more successful community integration. A leisure assessment should incorporate such areas as previous and current participation patterns, social interaction skills, knowledge of available leisure resources, attitude and activity skills, etc. Identification of individual preferences allows us to identify specific interests or hobbies, that may be natural motivators to make the attainment of objectives and goals an enjoyable and successful experience for clients. One of the most common approaches used to identify interests is the use of interest inventories.

Each of these areas, general functioning, leisure functioning and preference identification, examines a separate and distinct component. Together, these assessments provide critical information related to client abilities, needs and personal interests. It is important that the therapeutic recreation assessment process address each of these three areas to help practitioners more fully understand the impact of a client's functional ability on their leisure, and to better work with a client to assist them in optimizing their abilities and lead a life that is personally satisfying and meaningful. It is not acceptable, as is many times the case, for therapeutic recreation practitioners to address only one of these particular areas, without also considering the impact of the other two on client functioning (Figure 3). At present a very limited number of rigorously tested assessment instruments are available specifically for use in therapeutic recreation. For the assessment of general functioning, assessment instruments are often borrowed from other professions for use in therapeutic recreation. These borrowed instruments do not relate specifically to leisure; they focus on functional performance. To assess leisure functioning the therapeutic recreation professional has often found it necessary to develop an assessment tool at the agency level for personal use. Often these agency-specific assessment tools are not tested due to the time and energy involved in the testing process. The absence of appropriately designed and validated instruments has left the therapeutic recreation practitioner with limited options in selecting and using assessments in program planning. This is the most critical area for the profession if we are to demonstrate our unique and independent contribution to health service provision.

Linking Assessment to Outcome

The link between assessment and outcome is, of course, the therapeutic intervention. The important issue here is to link specific interventions for specific problems, with specific outcomes. Much research is needed before the assessment results can be used to choose a strategy for success. But this research is necessary if the profession is to develop on a scientific basis.

A critical part of the intervention is the integration of the available information and the formulation of a plan. The information required for such a formulation must contain measures of cognitive, affective and psycho-motor domains of the client (Table 3), set against the demands of the task(s) or goal(s) and the expected gains through intervention. Choosing a leisure goal based only on preferences selected from a menu of relatively undemanding activities (rather than setting individualized goals to be met through therapeutic recreation intervention) is inadequate. Such activity focused programs are sometimes seen in long-term care institutions. For the client to participate in personally meaningful and satisfying activities, these activities must to some degree match the preferences *and abilities* of the client, and perhaps include an element of challenge. On the other hand, the activity must be realistic. Adequate functional ability to meet the challenge of the activity is necessary otherwise frustration ensues. It is a measure of the skills of the therapeutic recreation professional, and indeed of the therapy team as a whole, that a realistic goal of interest is selected and that the necessary functional ability, knowledge and specific leisure skills are developed as the client moves toward successful achievement of the goal. Furthermore, the skillful therapeutic recreation professional will involve both the client and family in the goal setting process and ensure that the client acquires a sense of achievement as the program progresses. The achievement of defined milestones on the way to the goal maintains client motivation and participation.

> *"The easiest thing in the world is to have the client come to a program for the first time . . . . . the hardest is to ensure that the client will return, to take part again."* Dr. Fred Humphrey

The Importance of Goal Setting and Goal Achievement

Client assessment, particularly in older adults, can identify many problems; indeed at times the list can seem endless and the challenge overwhelming. Defining client goals helps to make clear the relative importance of various strengths and limitations of the client. Goals can range from the achievement of a simple task to major lifestyle changes. Goal setting and monitoring of goal achievement, along with clearly defined therapeutic recreation intervention, are key components of the outcome measurement process. Goal setting serves many important functions. For example, goal setting (1) defines the areas of concern and the functional and behavioural underpinnings of the problem requiring intervention; (2) unifies the client and team members in their direction and efforts; (3) permits prioritization of activities, through clear identification of the area of concern; and this in turn allows a reality check; is the goal realistic?; (4) permits reappraisal of activity over time; is the goal getting closer?; and (5) allows future planning to begin.

Goal statements should be realistic and concisely written. Goal statements should:

- ❑ expect change in client behaviour
- ❑ specify client behaviour that can be measured
- ❑ be achievable during the client's present length of involvement in the service
- ❑ take into consideration the discharge prognosis of the client
- ❑ clearly specify time line expectations for reaching the goal
- ❑ express goals which are mutually established with, and agreed upon by, the client and/or their family

Measuring Outcomes

Specific outcomes should derive from defined interventions. The impact of specific programs can be evaluated by measuring change, over time, in client functioning or behaviour.[3,33] It is important to measure client progress at several different times during their program or intervention to determine when the most change occurs and when further intervention or treatment has a minimal effect. Outcome information will help therapeutic recreation professionals to better understand what types of clients respond best to different types of therapeutic recreation treatment or intervention and what goals are realistic for them.

Specifically, outcomes related to client functioning in leisure or therapeutic recreation are used for, and will help to: (1) evaluate the effectiveness of certain types of intervention or services; (2) allow therapeutic recreation professionals to compare different types of interventions and approaches; (3) provide valuable information to better help allocate limited or scarce resources; (4) guide program planning for the future; and (5) encourage innovative approaches in areas where improvement can or cannot be demonstrated. Outcome information is now required by accrediting bodies such as CARF, JCAHO, CCHSA and third party funders, as well as by administrators in most facilities or agencies.

Outcomes are usually measured in one of two ways, either through change or gain scores or the achievement of goals. These methods are not totally distinct. For example, a goal can be expressed in terms of the amount of change in a particular sphere (gain score) needed to achieve it. To measure outcomes using change or gain scores, an appropriate standardized instrument is selected and utilized to measure change, over time, in the functioning or behaviour that one would expect to change as a result of the intervention provided. Monitoring times may vary depending upon the setting within which the therapeutic recreation practitioner works. For example, if a practitioner employed in a long-term care setting wants to gauge client functioning or client response to specific programs or intervention, progress might be monitored and recorded monthly. On the other hand, therapeutic recreation practitioners working in very clinically active units with short lengths of stay would monitor and document more often, possibly weekly. The LCM provides therapeutic recreation practitioners working in a variety of settings with one means of documenting change, over time, related to leisure functioning.

> *". . . learning is directly proportional to the amount of fun one is having."*
> Robert Pike

> *". . . success of intervention cannot always be measured in terms of physical recovery."*
> Kemp, Brummel-Smith and Ramsdell

The setting and achievement of goals allows the therapeutic recreation practitioner, team, client and family to evaluate the success, or lack of success, of the (therapeutic) programs. As mentioned, goals are client-centred and ideally impact positively on quality of life. Not all goals are achieved. Sometimes new insights into the clients abilities only become clear through working with the client in a therapeutic setting. For example, cognition may prove to be more impaired than initially thought, or motivation less than expected. In such cases goals need to be revised. Even when things go well, not all goals are accomplished. Generally speaking, if all goals are met all the time, they are being set too low. Similarly, recurrent failure implies the goals are routinely set too high. Even with the most skillful goal-setting team, goals can be missed or surpassed.

It is relatively simple to turn the degree of goal achievement into a score that, when amalgamated across clients, provides a measure of program success. There are several ways to do this. For example, and at the simplest level, goals can simply be recorded as achieved or not. The overall success of the program can be stated as the percentage of goals which have been achieved. Goal attainment scaling is a more sophisticated technique for measuring the

FIGURE 4. DOCUMENTATION CYCLE IN THERAPEUTIC RECREATION

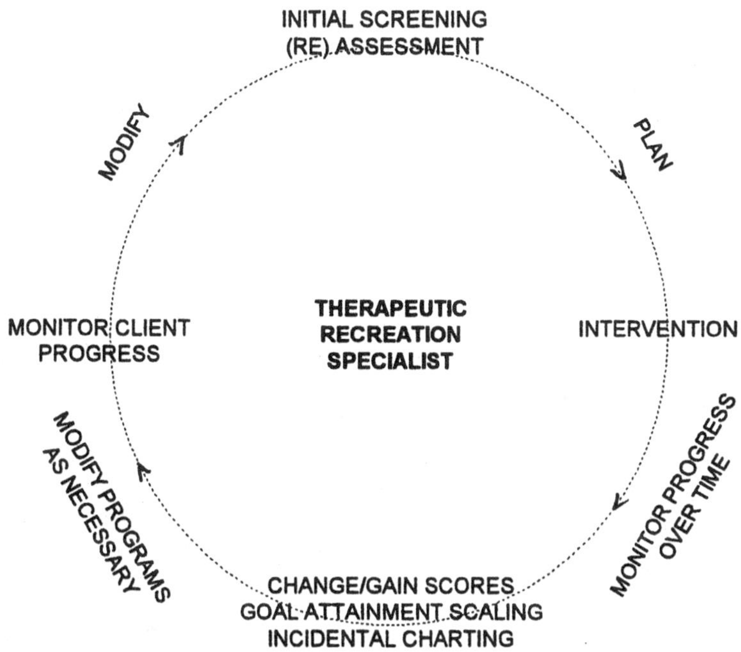

degree of goal attainment. With this method the team not only sets the goals but defines goals which are one and two steps above and below the target goal, thereby creating an individualized 5-point scale (ranging from -2 to +2) for each goal. The methods of scoring the attainment scale, and of amalgamating several goals into one score are discussed in Chapter 4. More detailed information regarding the use of goal attainment scaling in therapeutic recreation can be found in Chapter 4.

Clients and Settings

All therapeutic recreation practitioners must carry out client assessments, set goals, monitor client progress and measure outcomes. No matter the setting or population with whom therapeutic recreation practitioners work, each of our clients can be described as falling into one of the following three distinct categories:

We work with clients to:

1. improve levels of physical, cognitive, affective and/or social function
2. maintain current levels of physical, cognitive, affective and/or social function
3. minimize decrease in physical, cognitive, affective and/or social function

For example, those clients with whom therapeutic recreation practitioners are working on *improving* functioning are typically found in rehabilitation settings; those with whom practitioners are working on *maintaining* functional levels are usually found in longer stay or long-term care settings; and those clients with whom practitioners are working to *minimize a decrease in* functioning are generally found on specialized units (e.g., Alzheimer's Unit; Special Care Unit; etc.). The latter are clients who cannot help but deteriorate due to the progression of the disease process (e.g., dementia). However, it is important for therapeutic recreation practitioners to work with these clients to ensure that they have the opportunity to function at the optimal level of their *limited* level of functioning, thereby possibly slowing the curve of their decline. In each of these cases it is critically important for therapeutic recreation practitioners to be fully aware of their clients' physical and cognitive functioning capabilities, leisure functioning capabilities, as well as individual interests and preferences. This information must be captured as part of the assessment process and change in this functioning must be objectively and routinely documented over time.

". . . individuals require sufficient pleasurable experiences to outweigh whatever painful ones exist in daily life."
Kemp, Brummel-Smith and Ramsdell

". . .the greatest essentials to happiness in this life are something to do, something to love and something to hope for."
Joseph Addison

Conclusion

Measuring outcomes, and providing better documentation in general (Figure 4), has become critically important for all allied health professions, including therapeutic recreation. Of particular importance are the long-term outcomes following discharge, that allow health professionals and funders to determine how successful interventions were in enabling clients to live as independently as possible once they have returned home. Outcome information will assist all therapeutic recreation professionals in justifying the type, frequency and length of intervention necessary for achieving optimal results.

All therapeutic recreation practitioners must take responsibility for, and make a commitment to, ensuring that change in leisure functioning of their clients is objectively measured and routinely incorporated into their daily therapeutic recreation practice.

References

1. Anthony, W.A. & Farkas, M. (1982). A client outcome planning model for assessing psychiatric rehabilitation interventions. Schizophrenia Bulletin, 8, 13-38.

2. Brown, M., Gordon, W.A. & Piller, L. (19983). Functional assessment and outcome measurement: An integrative review. Annual Review of Rehabilitation, 3, 93-120.

3. Fuhrer, M.J. (1987). Overview of outcome analysis in rehabilitation. In M.J. Fuhrer (Ed.), Rehabilitation Outcomes: Analysis and Measurement (pp. 1-15). Baltimore: Paul H. Brookes.

4. Johnston, M.V., Keith, R.A. & Hinderer, S.R. (1992). Measurement standards for interdisciplinary medical rehabilitation. Archives of Physical Medicine and Rehabilitation, 73, S-3-S-23.

5. Kemp, R., Brummel-Smith, K. & Ramsdell, J.W. (1990). Geriatric rehabilitation. Boston: College-Hill.

6. Nosek, M.A. (1987). Outcome analysis in independent living. In M.J. Fuhrer (Ed.), Rehabilitation Outcomes: Analysis and Measurement (pp. 71-83). Baltimore: Paul H. Brookes.

7. Piper, M.C. (1992). Rehabilitation outcome measures: Where do we go from here? Canadian Journal of Public Health, 83, S-69-S-70.

8. Arnold, S.B. (1991). Measurement of quality of life in the frail elderly. In J.E. Birren, J.E. Lubben, J.C. Rowe & D.E. Deutchman (Eds.), The Concept of Measurement of Quality of Life in the Frail Elderly (pp. 50-73). New York: Academic Press.

9. The National Advisory Council on Aging. (1993). Policy paper no. 13 on Canada's Oldest Seniors: Maintaining the Quality of Their Lives, Ottawa, Ontario.

10. Brummel-Smith, K. (1993). Research in rehabilitation. Clinics in Geriatric Medicine, 9(4), 895-904.

11. Smith, I. (1994). Research moves out of the ivory tower. Rehabilitation Management, 62-64.

12. Forer, S. (1987). Outcome analysis for program service management. In M.J. Fuhrer (Ed.), Rehabilitation Outcomes: analysis and Measurement (pp. 115-136).

13. DeJong, G., & Hughes, J. (1982). Independent living methodology for measuring long-term outcomes. Archives of Physical Medicine and Rehabilitation, 63, 68-73.

14. Birren, J.E., Lubben, J.E., Rowe, J.C. & Deutchman, D.E. (Eds.) (1991). The concept of measurement of quality of life in the frail elderly. New York: Academic Press.

15. DeJong, G. (1987). Medical rehabilitation outcome measurement in a changing health care market. In M.J. Fuhrer (Ed.), Rehabilitation Outcomes: Analysis and Measurement (pp. 261-271). Baltimore: Paul H. Brookes.

16. Kloseck, M., Crilly, R.G., Ellis, G.D. & Lammers, E. (1996). Leisure Competence Measure: Development and reliability testing of a scale to measure functional outcomes in therapeutic recreation. Therapeutic Recreation Journal, 30(1), 13-26.

17. American Psychological Association. (1974). Standards for educational and psychological tests. Washington, D.C.: Author.

18. Carmines, E.G. & Zeller, R.A. (1979). Reliability and validity assessment. Newbury Park: Sage.

19. Bartz. A.E. (1988). Basic statistical concepts. New York: MacMillan.

20. Gay, L.R. (1992). Educational research. New York: MacMillan.

21. Creswell, J.W. (1994). Research design: Qualitative & quantitative approaches. California: Sage.

22. Silva, F. (1993). Psychometric foundations and behavioral assessment. California: Sage.

23. Peterson, C.A. & Gunn, S.L. (1984). Therapeutic recreation program design: Principles and procedures. New Jersey: Prentice-Hall.

24. Datillo, J. & Murphy, W.D. (1991). Leisure education program planning: A systematic approach. Pennsylvania, Venture.

25. Dowd, E.T. (Ed.) (1984). Leisure counselling: Concepts and applications. Illinois: Charles C. Thomas.

26. Studenski, S. & Duncan, P.W. (1993). Measuring rehabilitation outcomes. Clinics in Geriatric Medicine, 9(4), 823-830.

27. Kloseck, M. & Crilly, R.G. (in progress). Leisure Competence Measure: Measuring outcomes in therapeutic recreation.

28. Cohen, B.F., Ridley, D.E. & Cohen, M.R. (1985). Teaching skills to psychiatric disabled persons. In H.A. Marlowe Jr. & R.B. Weinberg (Eds.), Competence development: Theory and practice in special populations (pp. 118-145). Illinois: Charles C. Thomas.

29. Ford, M.E. (1985). The concept of competence: Themes and variations. In H.A. Marlowe Jr. & R.B. Weinberg (Eds.), Competence development: Theory and practice in special populations (pp. 3-49). Illinois: Charles C. Thomas.

30. Norris, N. (1991). The trouble with competence. Cambridge Journal of Education, 21(3), 331-341.

31. Sternberg, R.J. & Kolligen, J. (1990). Competence considered. Yale Press.

32. Wagner, K.A. (1987). Outcome analysis in comprehensive medical rehabilitation. In M.J. Fuhrer (Ed.), Rehabilitation Outcomes: Analysis and Measurement (pp. 19-28). Baltimore: Paul H. Brookes.

33. Stumbo, N.J. (1996). A proposed accountability model for therapeutic recreation services. Therapeutic Recreation Journal, 30(4), 246-259.

34. Stolee, P., Rockwood, K., Fox, R.A. & Streiner, D.L. (1992). The use of goal attainment scaling in a geriatric care setting. Journal of the American Geriatrics Society, 40, 574-578.

35. Kiresuk, Smith & Cardillo (1994). Goal attainment scaling: Application, theory and measurement. New Jersey: Lawrence Erlbaum.

Additional Resources

Spector, P.E. (1992). Summated rating scale construction: An introduction. California: Sage.

DeVellis, R.F. (1991). Scale development: Theory and applications. California: Sage.

Huck, S.W., Cormier, W.H. & Bounds, W.G. (1974). Reading statistics and research. New York: Harper & Row.

Liebert, R.M. & Liebert, L.L. (1995). Science and behavior: An introduction to methods of psychological research. New Jersey, Prentice-Hall.

Linn, R.L. (Ed.). (1993). Educational measurement. Arizona: Orynx Press.

Malkin, M.J. & Howe, C.Z. (Eds.) (1993). Research in therapeutic recreation: Concepts and methods. Pennsylvania: Venture.

Suen, H.K. (1990). Principles of test theories. New Jersey: Lawrence Erlbaum.

McDowell, I. & Newell, C. (1987). Measuring health: A guide to rating scales and questionnaires. New York: Oxford.

CHAPTER 2

Theoretical Frameworks and Conceptualization of the LCM

SUMMARY

- *In order to further build the body of knowledge related to therapeutic recreation and help other allied health professionals to better understand the role and "fit" of therapeutic recreation as part of the overall health care delivery system, it is important and necessary to link therapeutic recreation practice and research to broader conceptual and theoretical frameworks.*

- *Social psychological theories, theories related to aging and theories of disability may provide therapeutic recreation practitioners with a helpful framework for guiding future research efforts.*

- *Three major disability frameworks are the World Health Organization's classification system, Nagi's model used by the U.S. National Academy of Sciences Institute of Medicine and the National Center for Medical Rehabilitation Research framework, National Institute of Health in the United States.*

- *The World Health Organization's classification system, the leisure-based philosophy for therapeutic recreation operationalized through the Leisure Ability Model, and behavioural constructs of competence outlined in social and gerontological literature form the theoretical basis of the LCM*

Chapter 2
Theoretical Frameworks and Conceptualization of the LCM

Introduction

One of the major concerns outlined in the literature is that much of the research and many papers published in therapeutic recreation lack conceptual and theoretical frameworks.[1,2,3,4,5,27] For example Stumbo,[3] while investigating knowledge required for therapeutic recreation practice, discovered that there was very little interest in, or attention given to, theory and philosophy of practice in therapeutic recreation. "Theories and philosophies of therapeutic recreation" and "theories on philosophies of play, leisure and recreation" , in terms of their importance, were rated 15th and 27th out of 37 content areas. Likewise, Bedini and Wu[2] reviewed research published in the *Therapeutic Recreation Journal* from 1986 to 1990 and discovered that a mere 26% of the all articles published were grounded in, or made reference to, theoretical or conceptual frameworks. Ellis[5] and Sylvester[4] argue that therapeutic recreation does not have "theory" or a "rigorous philosophical base" compared to other professions. For a profession seeking to increase status and gain credibility in inter-disciplinary health settings, this is disappointing. It is absolutely critical that therapeutic recreation research is linked to conceptual and theoretical constructs and that therapeutic recreation professionals make a serious effort to ensure that existing theoretical and conceptual frameworks are used to guide their research.

Shank, Coyle, Boyd and Kinney[1] argue that "sharing a common framework could foster more collaborative and interdisciplinary research" (p. 190). These authors propose a modified conceptual model of disability (based on a framework developed by the National Center for Medical Rehabilitation Research in the United States) that might be useful for therapeutic recreation practitioners in medical rehabilitation settings. It is critical that theories, whether they are social science theories, theories related to aging or disability theories, are linked directly with leisure, and more importantly, linked to the applied needs of therapeutic recreation practitioners. In order to best provide a service to the public, an understanding of human development and behaviour, as well as an understanding of the underlying theoretical foundations of leisure and leisure behaviour, is absolutely necessary. Often, even if considered important, therapeutic recreation, when weighed against other priorities (particularly during a time of significant restructuring and funding constraints), ends up being compromised or being subsumed within other health-related professions. To better help others understand the unique contribution of therapeutic recreation, to demonstrate outcomes related to therapeutic recreation intervention, and to lead the advancement of measuring psychosocial outcomes in general, all therapeutic recreation practitioners must begin to link their work, research and publications to broader conceptual and theoretical frameworks. Atheoretical research is no longer acceptable.

The subsequent sections briefly highlight some common social psychological theories, theories associated with aging and conceptualizations of disability and competence that may be helpful to therapeutic recreation practitioners. The purpose is to make professionals aware of existing theoretical and conceptual frameworks that have direct relevance to therapeutic recreation and may be drawn on for support. There are many excellent books available outlining each of these theories in detail; these are referenced at the end of this chapter. Two books that professionals might find particularly helpful are: (1) *Social Psychology of Leisure* by Mannell and Kleiber[6]; and (2) *Handbook of Psychology and Aging* by Birren and Schaie.[7]

Social Psychological Theories

The belief that leisure may have the potential to significantly impact health and well-being stems from the underlying concepts of perceived freedom, intrinsic and extrinsic motivation, and locus of control.[8] From a social psychological perspective an experience is considered to be leisure when an individual perceives themselves as having the ability and being free to take part in those things that are personally meaningful and satisfying, and being able to exercise some control over their lives. This is a particularly important concept for the elderly many of whom, due to normal physiological decline and multiple losses with advancing age, become increasingly dependent on others (i.e., have external loci of control).

> **Practice Point:**
>
> It must be an underlying tenet of any therapeutic endeavour that an individual's degree of control be maximized.

Major social psychological theories that describe how leisure may impact health and well-being that may be drawn upon include attribution theory,[9] motivation theory,[10,11,12,13] self-determination theory,[14] self-efficacy theory,[15.16] locus of control theory,[17] learned helplessness,[18] theory of substitutability,[9] theory of flow,[19] the recreation and relaxation theory described by Ellis[20] and Neulinger[8] similar to the pleasure, relaxation and fun theory described by Mannell and Kleiber,[6] and Lazarus' theory of stress and coping.[23]

For example, attribution theory[9] examines the relationship between leisure, personality and situational forces. This theory suggests that behaviour is caused by individual dispositional attributes as well as situational or environmental attributes. In addition to influencing behaviour, these attributes may also have a psychological impact. Iso-Ahola[9] provides the following example. In a certain circumstance, "if a person attributes his failure to bad luck rather than to the lack of his ability, he is then likely to persist in and continue his activity instead of giving up" (p. 185). This provides a coping mechanism for the individual and affords a means by which they are able to preserve their self-esteem in the event of failure in a specific task.

Motivation theory examines internal and external forces and the impact of these forces on individual behaviour. Motivation has been studied in a variety of ways. One very influential approach has been to conceptualize the construct of motivation as internal needs that drive or promote behaviours that will satisfy those needs. For example, Maslow[12] describes hierarchically ordered human needs ranging from basic physiological needs, to esteem needs, and ultimately the need for self-actualization. Maslow[12] argues that once existing needs are met, individuals continually strive to reach their fullest potential (self-actualization). White[13] and Harter[11] suggest that all individuals have a need to feel competent, that this need motivates behaviour and that successful interaction with one's environment and the resulting feelings of pleasure are critical factors in this process. Likewise, Deci and Ryan[14] link self-determination to intrinsic motivation, emphasizing the notions of control and choice.

Self-efficacy theory[15,16] suggests that the perceived self-efficacy of an individual influences the individual's behaviour and directly impacts the effort the individual will expend and the length of time they will persist in any given activity.

Practice Point:

Low motivation in a rehabilitation setting may be a result of clinical depression and all team members should be aware of this as a possibility.

Low motivation inhibits progress toward goals.

Motivation may differ for different tasks.

The learned helplessness theory[18] suggests that if an individual believes a situation to be uncontrollable, feelings of helplessness will result. Similarly, if an individual believes that their actions or behaviour will make no difference in a given situation, the likelihood of the individual exhibiting those actions or behaviours will decrease. Learned helplessness has been associated with depression and this theory supports the importance of perceived control in the lives of individuals.

Substitutability theory[9] "addresses the factors that influence one's willingness and tendency to substitute original leisure behaviour when the need for substitution has arisen" (p. 370). It is suggested that the act of substituting is a "psychological process" (p. 367) and that an individual's openness to alternatives depends upon why the substitution was necessary, as well as other options available to the individual. A central tenet of this theory is perceived choice and freedom. This is commonly needed when old leisure pursuits are no longer possible.

Practice Point:

In practice the client may require a period of adjustment before he/she is ready to pursue an alternative activity in lieu of chosen activities.

Consistent with the belief that freedom of choice and intrinsic motivation are necessary to experience leisure, and that leisure experiences are influenced by both personal and social factors, the theory of flow[19] focuses on an individual's subjective experience of leisure and the resulting effect of those experiences on the individual. Key concepts of this theory are: (1) that an individual's leisure experience will vary in intensity; (2) that individuals will differ in their intensity and experience; (3) a leisure experience is mediated by cognitive and affective attributes; and (4) a leisure experience and an individual's awareness of it are transient.

Recreation and relaxation theory described by Ellis[20] and Neulinger[8] suggests that recreation provides an opportunity for relaxation and time away from work. This is similar to the pleasure, relaxation and fun theory proposed by Mannell and Kleiber[6] that describes enjoyment and pleasure as important components derived from leisure experience. Mannell and Kleiber suggest that these intermittent pleasurable experiences may, over time, contribute to individual well-being. During the past decade, with the shift in perspective from treatment of disease to a greater focus on physical and mental health and well-being of individuals, these theories may provide therapeutic recreation practitioners with a framework for guiding future research efforts.

Practice Point:

Many therapeutic recreation professionals are intuitively aware of the importance of self-determination and choice, as well as the obstructive effect of low motivation, lack of self-efficacy and a sense of helplessness. These concepts must be incorporated within the overall approach to therapeutic recreation intervention (see Figure 5).

Theories Associated with Aging

A number of theories exist to help examine psychological, social and environmental factors, the interactions of these factors and their subsequent impact on the behaviour of the elderly.

For example, Lawton and Nahemows' Competence and Environmental Press Theory[21] suggests that a particular level of ability is associated with competence and that individuals who experience more losses or declines will be less able to cope with environmental factors. Kahana's Congruence Model[22] suggests that individuals vary in their needs and that environments differ in their ability to satisfy these needs. This model is important when an individual's options are limited (i.e., institutionalization occurs). The model suggests that individual differences (e.g., living arrangements; personal needs; etc.) are important considerations when planning interventions. If at all possible the environment should be matched to the personal needs of the individual. Lazarus' theory of Stress and Coping[23] suggests that individuals evaluate their situations and determine potential "threats". Individuals then engage coping mechanisms in response to the perceived "threat". It has been argued that the presence of social support systems may affect an individual's perception of their situation and assessment of this needs to be part of any therapeutic recreation assessment.

Pastalam's Loss-Continuum Concept[24] suggests that growing older is associated with a series of losses that limit level of engagement. Losses increase with age and this results in a reduced ability to fully participate in society. The home and immediate personal environment of the individual then becomes most important. This should be taken into consideration when planning interventions or considering environmental changes.

Activity theory[25] suggests a positive relationship between engagement in activities and life satisfaction or successful aging in the elderly. Continuity theory[26] presumes activity, behaviour and personality patterns developed during one's early childhood years are related to patterns in later adult years. It is suggested that stability over the lifespan contributes to successful aging.

Practice Point:

It is important to examine previous lifestyle and engagement patterns of individuals as part of the overall therapeutic recreation assessment process.

Theoretical Frameworks of Disability

There appear to be three major conceptual frameworks of disability: (1) the World

Health Organization classification system;[28] (2) Nagi's model used by the U.S. National Academy of Sciences Institute of Medicine;[38,39] and (3) the National Center for Medical Rehabilitation Research framework, U.S. National Institute of Health.[1,40] Both the World Health Organization (WHO) model and Nagi's model recognize the influence of social and environmental factors on individuals with disabilities.

The WHO model operationalizes rehabilitation theory through the International Classification of Impairment, Disability and Handicap[28] and is a model that emphasizes the importance of social, attitudinal and environmental influences for individuals with disabilities. The WHO requires that outcomes are measured on the following three levels: (1) *Impairment* at the "organ system level"; (2) *Disability* as the "functional consequences of impairment"; and (3) *Handicap* as the "social and societal consequences of impairment and disability".[28] While there is international acceptance and wide usage of the WHO model, it does have some limitations. For example, much concern has been expressed over the term "handicap". This model was originally developed as a means of classifying the "consequences of diseases" and is now in the process of being revised by the WHO to better reflect broader definitions of health.[28] Nagi's model does not include a classification system. Similar to the WHO conceptualization of disability, this conceptual framework includes the concepts of "pathology", "impairment", "functional limitation" and "disability"[39]

The National Center for Medical Research framework developed by the National Institute of Health builds on the WHO and Nagi frameworks by incorporating "societal limitations" as a distinct piece of the disabling process.[1] Shank, Coyle, Boyd and Kinney[1] modified the National Center for Medical Research's conceptualization of disability to guide therapeutic recreation research. Readers wishing more detailed information on any of these models should consult either the World Health Organization's International Classification System of Impairment, Disability and Handicap,[28] Nagi's work,[38,39] the work of Pope and Tarlov[40] or the paper by Shank, Coyle, Boyd and Kinney[1] referenced at the end of this chapter.

The Concept of Competence

The concept of competence has been widely debated in the literature. It is a multifaceted construct for which researchers have had difficulty reaching consensus on interpretation and measurement. Most see this construct as a collection of skills and abilities which represent potential for action (behavioural possibilities).

Competencies therefore underlie, and are necessary antecedents of, optimal function. Some authors rank competencies hierarchically. For example Baltes[44,45] distinguished between basic competencies, needed for day to day living, and expanded competencies, needed for satisfying and meaningful living, which go beyond the competencies needed for simple existence. Expanded competence needs to be built on basic competencies. Nevertheless, the concept of competence and that of function are intertwined, given that the test of competence is the successful performance of a task. A fuller discussion of this area, with relevant references, can be found in the paper by Kloseck, Crilly, Ellis and Lammers.[35]

Much of the above finds relevance in therapeutic recreation practice, touching as it does on significant areas such as motivation, life satisfaction, self-efficacy, the ability to select new activities, etc. The LCM draws on some of these areas, particularly competence, disability and the leisure-based philosophy of practice as the theoretical basis of its development. Other aspects of these theories and concepts come into play in the operationalization of the LCM in practice (see Figure 5).

Conceptualization of the LCM

The LCM subscales were constructed according to: (1) rehabilitation theory operationalized through the International Classification of Impairment, Disability and Handicap (ICIDH) developed by the World Health Organization (WHO) in 1980;[28] (2) the behavioural construct of competence outlined in social and gerontological literature;[30,31,32,33,34,35] and (3) leisure education principles and the leisure-based philosophy for therapeutic recreation practice operationalized through the Leisure Ability Model.[29] For practical reasons the LCM was also designed to be consistent with the Functional Independence Measure (FIM),[41] a widely accepted and utilized instrument for outcome measurement in medical rehabilitation. This compatibility with the FIM affords therapeutic recreation practitioners, employed in health facilities using the FIM, a consistent and acceptable means of reporting at inter-disciplinary team conferences. The LCM also complies with the Commission on Accreditation for Rehabilitation Facilities (CARF), Joint Commission on Accreditation of Healthcare Organizations (JCAHO) and Canadian Council on Health Services Accreditation (CCHSA) standards. These accreditation standards require that outcome measures and evaluation systems address the accomplishment, or lack thereof, of functioning between admission and discharge, as well as the functional status of individuals at follow-up.[42,43] Fuhrer[27] argues that "ambiguities of interpretation (why change has occurred) can be minimized but not eliminated by choosing outcome variables

FIGURE 5. THERAPEUTIC RECREATION PROCESS DESIGNED TO OPTIMIZE CLIENT FUNCTIONING IN LEISURE

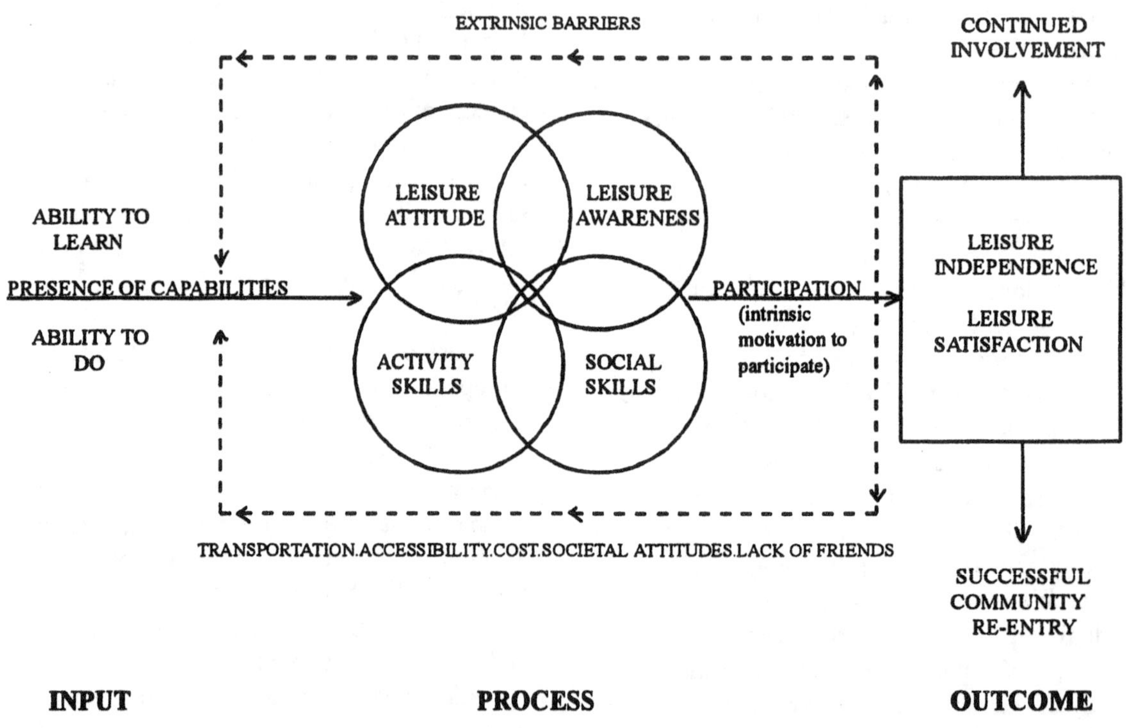

that are reasonably specific to the intervention being studied and by designing studies to neutralize the influence of factors other than the services provided" (p.4). The LCM subscales are specifically designed to address leisure education components (e.g., leisure attitude; leisure awareness; leisure skills; interpersonal skills; community integration; social contact; community participation) and leisure education outcomes identified and supported in leisure literature (Figure 5). The LCM subscales identify areas that can be targeted for defined interventions, leading to a specific type of outcome.

Rehabilitation Theory and the LCM

The ICIDH conceptualization of disability also provides a framework for the LCM. According to the ICIDH[28] *impairment* is considered any difficulty in "organ" functioning that results directly from illness. Impairment is defined as "any loss or abnormality of psychological, physiological or anatomical structure or function". *Disability* occurs at the "person" level and is defined as "any restriction or lack of ability resulting from an impairment" that interferes with everyday activity. This lack of ability may be temporary or permanent. This particular level is concerned with abilities and the focus is on education, training or adaptation techniques to allow clients to pursue an independent lifestyle that is personally meaningful and satisfying. *Handicap* is found at the "societal" level and is described as "a disadvantaged resulting from an impairment or disability that limits the fulfilment of a role

FIGURE 6. THE DIFFERENT DIMENSIONS OF THE CONSEQUENCES OF DISEASE AS DEFINED BY THE WORLD HEALTH ORGANIZATION (1980)

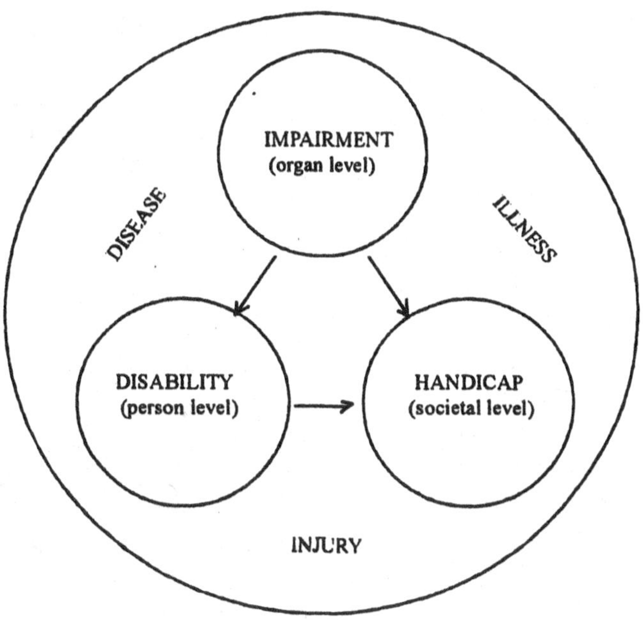

in society".[28] Fuhrer[27] argues that "the ICIDH affords a promising, albeit partial, foundation for a satisfactory theory of disablement and the rehabilitation process" (p. 13) through the constructs of impairment, disability and handicap.

The WHO model[28] emphasizes the importance of social, attitudinal and environmental influences on an individual with an impairment (Figure 6). In the context of the WHO classifications, needs at the level of disability and handicap are addressed predominantly by psychosocial services.[36,37] The LCM, in the context of WHO terminology, addresses the "disability" level by examining alterations in clients' abilities to function in their leisure. Efforts are primarily focused on providing education and adaptation techniques to allow clients to pursue an independent lifestyle through reduction in disability.

Competence and the LCM

Numerous conceptualizations of competence can be found in existing literature. The underlying conceptual framework of the LCM is consistent with the behavioural construct of competence that suggests individual competence is hierarchically arranged with increasing levels of complexity.[30,31,33,44,45] We have adopted the view that competencies are the underpinnings of function, those skills which prepare the individual for successful action. Part of the LCM, the first 6 subscales, concentrate on client capabilities and competencies required, whereas the remaining 2 subscales are designed to measure actual performance. The concept of competence extends from the acquisition of the basic essential skills through to their actual application in real-life situations. Therapeutic recreation professionals attempt to move the client from the acquisition of those skills to the achievement of successful, quality experiences.

Most measurement instruments used in health care environments, including the LCM, measure function under controlled situations to predict function in real-life situations, although at times field trips to directly evaluate the latter are possible. Additional information on the conceptualization of competence and the LCM may be found in the paper by Kloseck, Crilly, Ellis and Lammers.[35]

The Leisure-Based Philosophy for Therapeutic Recreation Practice and the LCM

The leisure-based philosophy for therapeutic recreation practice outlines a continuum through which an individual's ability may be optimized through the development of functional and leisure-related skills.[29,47] The central tenet of this philosophical approach is that one's ability to engage in personally meaningful and satisfying activities is dependent upon individual skills, knowledge and attitudes related to leisure.[29,47,48] The effect of leisure education on perceived competence of individuals has been demonstrated.[49,50,51]

The LCM identifies specific skills, knowledge and behaviour which individuals must posses in order to maximize independent and successful functioning in their leisure. Areas requiring improvement may then be identified through the LCM, mutually agreed upon with the clients and their families and then worked on to improve or develop behaviours necessary for more independent living and to ensure that individuals enjoy their leisure optimally. The LCM samples representative behaviours in eight leisure domains identified as necessary indicators of competence in leisure (Table 4).

TABLE 4. COMPONENTS OF THE LEISURE COMPETENCE MEASURE

LCM SUBSCALES	DESCRIPTION	TYPE OF MEASUREMENT
Leisure Awareness	Client's knowledge and understanding of leisure.	MEASURE OF CLIENT CAPABILITIES
Leisure Attitude	Behaviours exhibited and/or feelings demonstrated by the client which suggest attitude toward leisure involvement.	
Leisure Skills	Skills possessed by the client which affect leisure involvement.	
Cultural/Social Behaviours	Specific cultural/social behaviours exhibited by the client which affect his/her ability to function effectively in leisure activities.	
Interpersonal Skills	Client's ability to participate within various types of inter-individual and/or group situations.	
Community Integration Skills	Application of antecedent skills for successful involvement in community leisure activities.	
Social Contact	Type and duration of social contact the client has with others.	MEASURE OF CLIENT ACTUAL PERFORMANCE
Community Participation	Client's overall leisure participation pattern within the community.	

Therapeutic Recreation Assessment, Goal Setting and Intervention and the LCM

This section will explore how the LCM is applied in practice and also consider some simple important concepts of how, for example, to define a problem, prioritize intervention (i.e., what do we need to focus on?) and the concept of functional thresholds which have been found useful in thinking about functional loss and retrieval.

Functional independence requires ability that exceeds the demands of a specific task. Such ability does not in itself guarantee success as other factors also come into play, notably motivation and interest. Ability is not just physical but includes psychological and social components. The broader the function under consideration and the more the function involves quality of life and lifestyle factors, the broader the range of skills, abilities and resources required to achieve this level of function. Thus, independence in personal ADLs is less demanding than, for example, attending the theatre which requires skills in dressing, grooming, mobility, social appropriateness, hearing, vision, continence and so on.

Leisure, defining as it does a significant and varied segment of our lives makes broader and more complex demands on one's capacity. Any attempt to impact a client's function must be based on a full assessment of client strengths and limitations in relation to the task at hand. This in turn, requires a thorough assessment across relevant domains. The LCM categorizes and summarizes information related to the ability or disability of clients and the level of performance they are achieving. This allows therapeutic recreation professionals to identify areas of concern related to leisure functioning requiring attention through intervention. The purpose of therapeutic recreation intervention is to increase client independence, primarily by decreasing disability but also through task modification. Likewise, another important role of the therapeutic recreation professional is to work with communities to which their clients will be returning, as well as society as a whole, to reduce handicap (e.g., make facilities and programs more accessible; heighten public awareness of individuals with disabilities; decrease discrimination; etc.).

Following client assessment, a clear definition of goals helps to identify various strengths and areas of concern. Goals can range from fulfilling simple tasks to major lifestyle changes. The area of concern or problem, overall, then can be defined as the distance between a client's current level of function and that required by the goals. The role of therapeutic recreation intervention then becomes that of closing the distance. The problem can usually be subdivided into component functions and some of the general functional problems may fall into the area of competence of other disciplines. This both defines the need for a team approach and makes clear the critical functions to focus on, thereby increasing program efficiency. In many situations the therapeutic recreation professional does not work alone but alongside, in mutual interdependence, with other disciplines. Limitation to the independence that can be achieved with a client might necessitate the modification or simplification of the task(s) which forms the goal, the provision of aids or, finally, the provision of direct physical assistance.

The therapeutic recreation components of lifestyle goals established by the team or the therapeutic recreation professional alone, can be described in terms of functioning on the LCM. The difference between the abilities needed to achieve the goals and current function defines the problem for the therapeutic recreation professional and will serve as a reality check. Is the goal feasible? If not, then the goal needs to be reconsidered.

Thresholds of Function

Client independence changes over time, either improving as a result of recovery from illness or accident, or declining, perhaps rapidly as a result of an acute illness or injury, or slowly as occurs with age. A client's declining independence erodes functional ability, the most demanding functions going first. All function can be performed to varying degrees, at varying speeds and with varying degrees of success. Thus there is no well defined functional threshold above which one can, and below which one cannot, perform successfully. It is more like a broad zone, but for ease of discussion and illustration, we will consider it a clear threshold. Figure 7 illustrates the idea of the functional threshold, using mobility as an example.

The client shown has, through accumulation of the changes of age and perhaps some disease, declined in his functional independence. The client has reached a level of function still adequate for crossing the room, but not for running across a field. Although there is some decline in ability, social handicap is minimal. The next figure (Figure 8) illustrates the situation when the client gets ill and function declines rapidly. The stressor might be an acute injury as shown, or, especially in the elderly, a non-specific stressor such as a chest infection, a new sedating medication, and so on. This client has become dysfunctional and presents now with immobility and falling. Proper assessment and management will identify and remove or minimize the offending stressor if possible (e.g., stop the offending medication)

FIGURE 7. ILLUSTRATION OF A FUNCTIONAL THRESHOLD WITH THE SIMPLE ACTIVITY OF WALKING ACROSS A ROOM

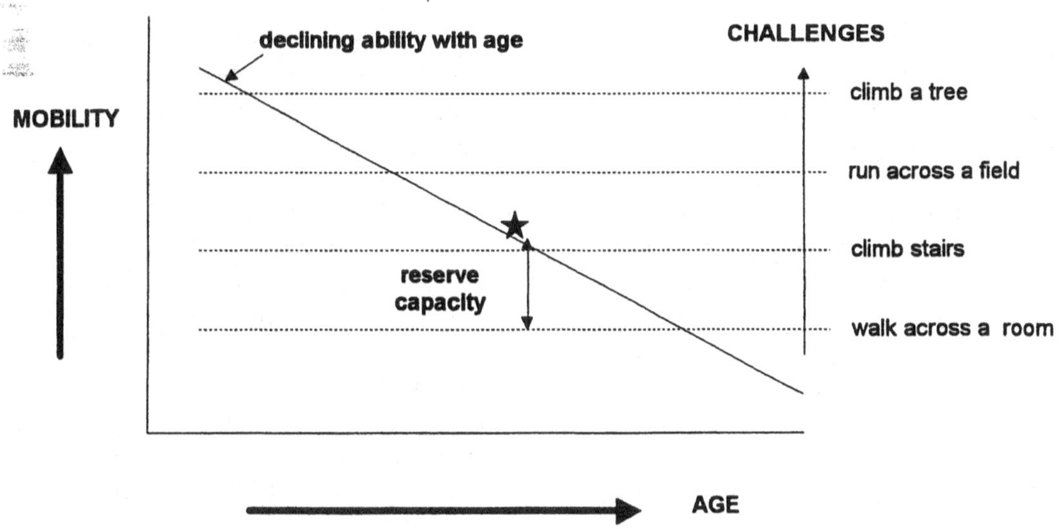

Note: The horizontal dotted lines define functional thresholds for the various examples given. Different activities are more or less demanding and the age-related decline in function eventually brings even well individuals below the thresholds for more demanding tasks. The star indicates the position of a person who can still safely walk across the room but for whom climbing the stairs is a borderline function.

FIGURE 8. ILLUSTRATION OF THE DECLINE IN FUNCTION WHEN A CLIENT GETS ILL AND FUNCTION DECLINES RAPIDLY

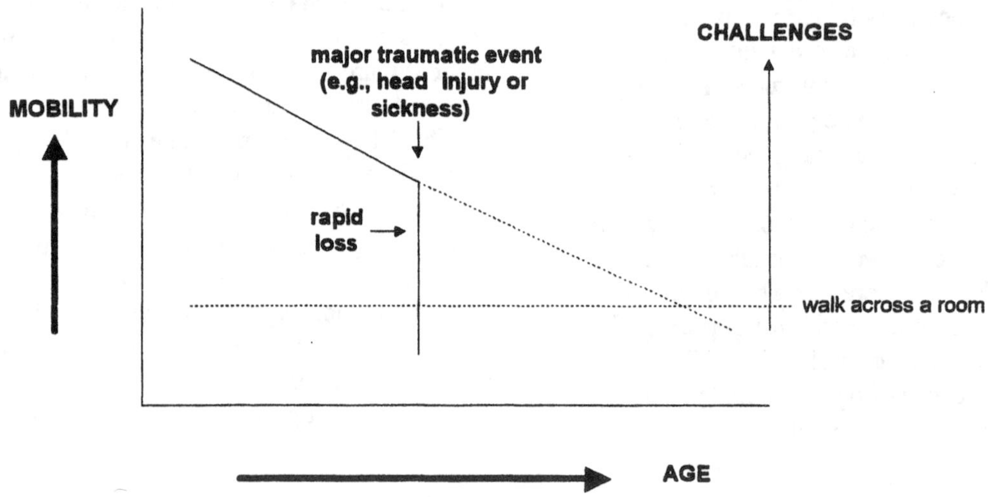

and hopefully allow the function to recover. Frequently, recovery is only partial, persistent damage remains and rehabilitation or treatment is necessary to minimize disability and handicap (Figure 8a).

Not uncommonly, especially in the elderly, dysfunction results from a series of smaller injuries and challenges, each eroding capacity or making the task more difficult. Thus mobility in the home can be compromised by shortness of breath from heart disease, pain from arthritic knees, poor footwear, muscle weakness from disuse, poor vision, poor lighting, cluttered rooms, etc., some of which erode client capacity and some increase task difficulty for the client. This is illustrated in Figure 9. The role of the team is to identify these multiple issues and resolve them, thereby helping the client to reclimb the steps in Figure 9, and also to identify ways of decreasing the difficulty of the task. The further the client gets above the threshold the greater the reserve will be and the more stable the achievement will prove.

The issue of mobility/immobility significantly impacts client functioning and quality of life, particularly for the elderly and therapeutic recreation professionals have a critical role to play in maximizing client functional capabilities *and maintaining* the client's level of functioning as much as possible. It is recognized that more successful outcomes can be achieved by blending the expertise of all professionals involved in a client's care. For example a physiotherapist, through intervention, may be able to improve a client's ability to walk but unless this ability is consistently and frequently practised and reinforced, this ability may be lost. Mobility and immobility (e.g., sitting; standing; transferring; lying; etc.) of clients also brings up important issues to consider when programming. Therapeutic recreation professionals, for example, must adjust program length, be aware of positioning and client tolerance during an activity. This, once again, reinforces the importance of a thorough and comprehensive assessment in order to set achievable client goals and plan programs geared to client abilities, needs and interests, as well as working collaboratively with interdisciplinary team members.

As can be seen, various activities present different levels of challenges. An individual's ability to perform an activity safely and successfully depends on how far above the level the client is. If the client is below the level they will be unable to perform the function (or will hurt themselves in attempting to do so). When the client falls below the level of function which is normally required for day to day living then a problem has occurred.

We have used mobility for illustration purposes but the same approach applies to many of the functions required for leisure involvement.

Where do Adaptive Aids Fit In?

Adaptive aids are simply ways of resolving the problem, closing the gap between the ability and the goal. Once again therapists may do this by either extending the client's ability, or making the task simpler such as occurs with walkers, reachers, card holders, modified fishing rods and reels, braces, wheelchairs, ramps, grab bars and so on (Figure 8b). Any remaining shortfall then needs to be bridged by the provision of assistance, which can either be intellectual, as in cueing, or physical assistance.

It is debatable whether the provision of aids should be considered to effectively reduce the independence of the client. We take the view that provided the client is independent in

FIGURE 8a. MAGNIFICATION OF PART OF FIGURE 8 TO SHOW SUBSEQUENT CLIENT PROGRESS

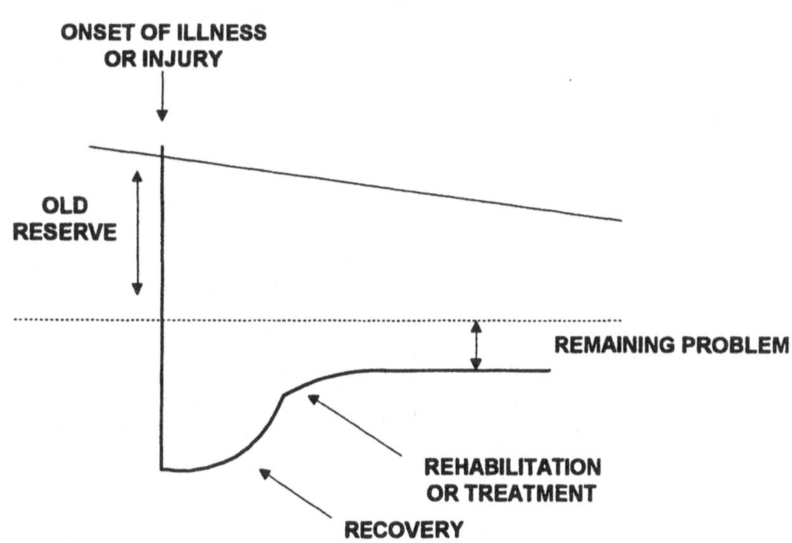

Note: Function improves as recovery proceeds and improves further with therapeutic intervention or rehabilitation. In this particular example the client is still below the threshold and hence limitations remain.

FIGURE 8b. EFFECT OF PROVISION OF AIDS AND ENVIRONMENTAL MODIFICATION

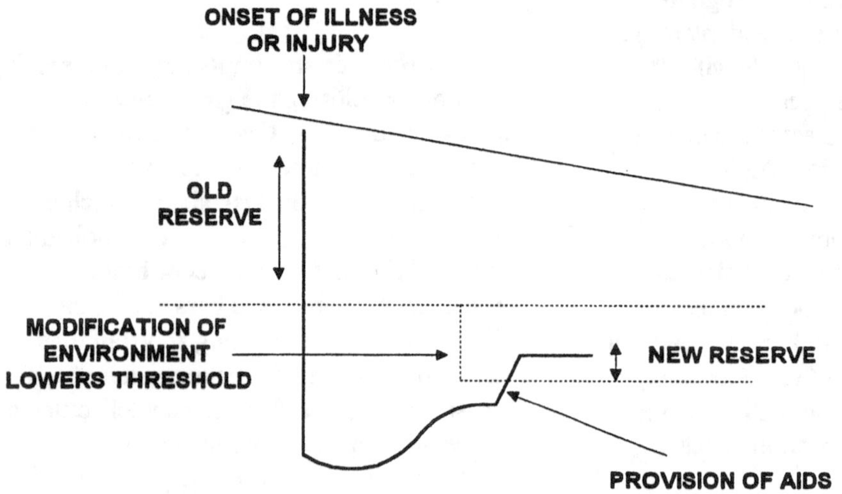

Note: The provision of aids has further improved function, and the modification of the environment has made the task less demanding. The client is now above the threshold and will be independent in the performance of this task, but with little reserve capacity.

FIGURE 9. EFFECT OF CUMULATIVE CHRONIC STRESSORS AND CHANGING ENVIRONMENTAL DEMANDS

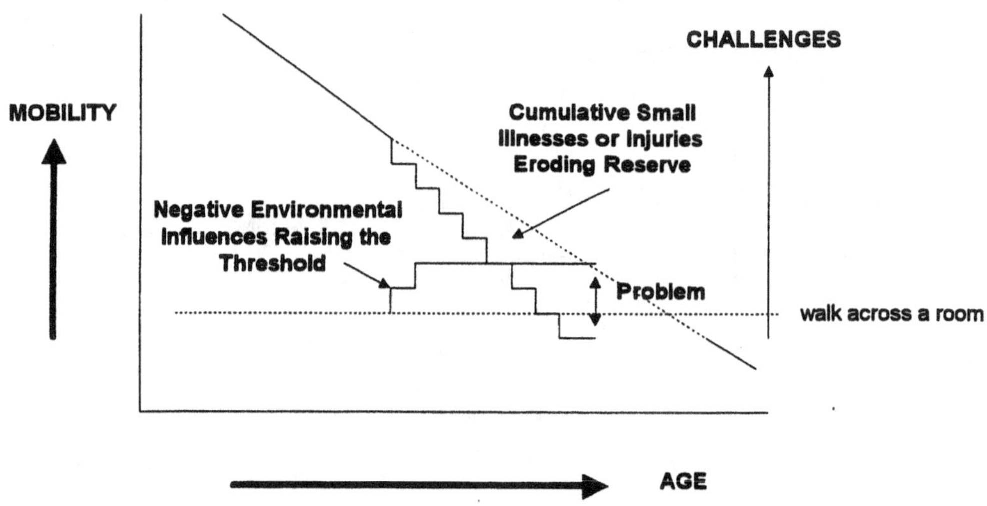

Note: A common situation with the elderly, in particular, is where the accumulation of chronic problems reduces ability and negative environmental change, such as might occur on moving to a new home, makes the task more difficult. The result is loss of function for this particular activity.

their use, then he or she is independent. We all use aids in our everyday life to extend our abilities, everything from cars to computers to can openers, without feeling any compromise of our abilities; indeed we view them as extending our abilities and our independence. Similar arguments can be made regarding environmental adaptations and this view becomes more defensible as society responds to the needs of individuals with disabilities and accessible environments become more common. Conceptually there is little difference between an elevator for the non-disabled and a ramp for individuals with a disability. It is true, however, that the more specialized the adaptation the more limited the (geographic) sphere of independence will be. Adaptive aids or equipment are common in therapeutic recreation practice and for the above reasons the LCM does not penalise for their use, provided the client is fully independent.

Points to Ponder. . .

. . . abilities and tasks are not dichotomous concepts but a continuous variable.

For example, does a walking aid, reacher, card holder, etc. extend an individual's ability or simplify a task?

Clients and Programs: From Theory to Practice

To this point various important theoretical and conceptual models relevant to therapeutic recreation have been reviewed. The following diagrams attempt to "pull it all together" by providing an overview of the whole process. This process is examined both from the point of view of the client and from the point of view of the program, introducing, in the latter case, the importance of program evaluation. Program evaluation will not be discussed, in depth, in this manual. However, references are provided at the end of this chapter for readers wishing to read further on this topic.[52,53,54,55,56]

Figure 10 lays out a brief diagrammatic representation of the overall process of assessment, goal setting, influencing factors, environmental modification and performance outcomes that have been touched on in previous sections. Figure 11 outlines in greater detail the process of therapeutic intervention, moving from the assessment in the three main domains discussed, through interpretation of the findings, goal setting and and planning, to short and long-term outcomes as they apply to a particular client. The concepts here are generic and will require personalization to the client's specific needs. Figure 11 also highlights were the LCM "fits" and is able to contribute to this process. Figure 12 outlines the process of therapeutic program functioning and evaluation. The therapeutic process, shown in Figure 11, is displayed horizontally, and the shaded boxes show examples of measures of program activity. Short and long-term outcomes are measures of program success. The measures of program activity are important for administrative and fiscal reasons, the measures of outcomes important for accountability and program survival.

FIGURE 10. OVERALL PROCESS LEADING FROM CLIENT ASSESSMENT TO SUCCESSFUL OUTCOME

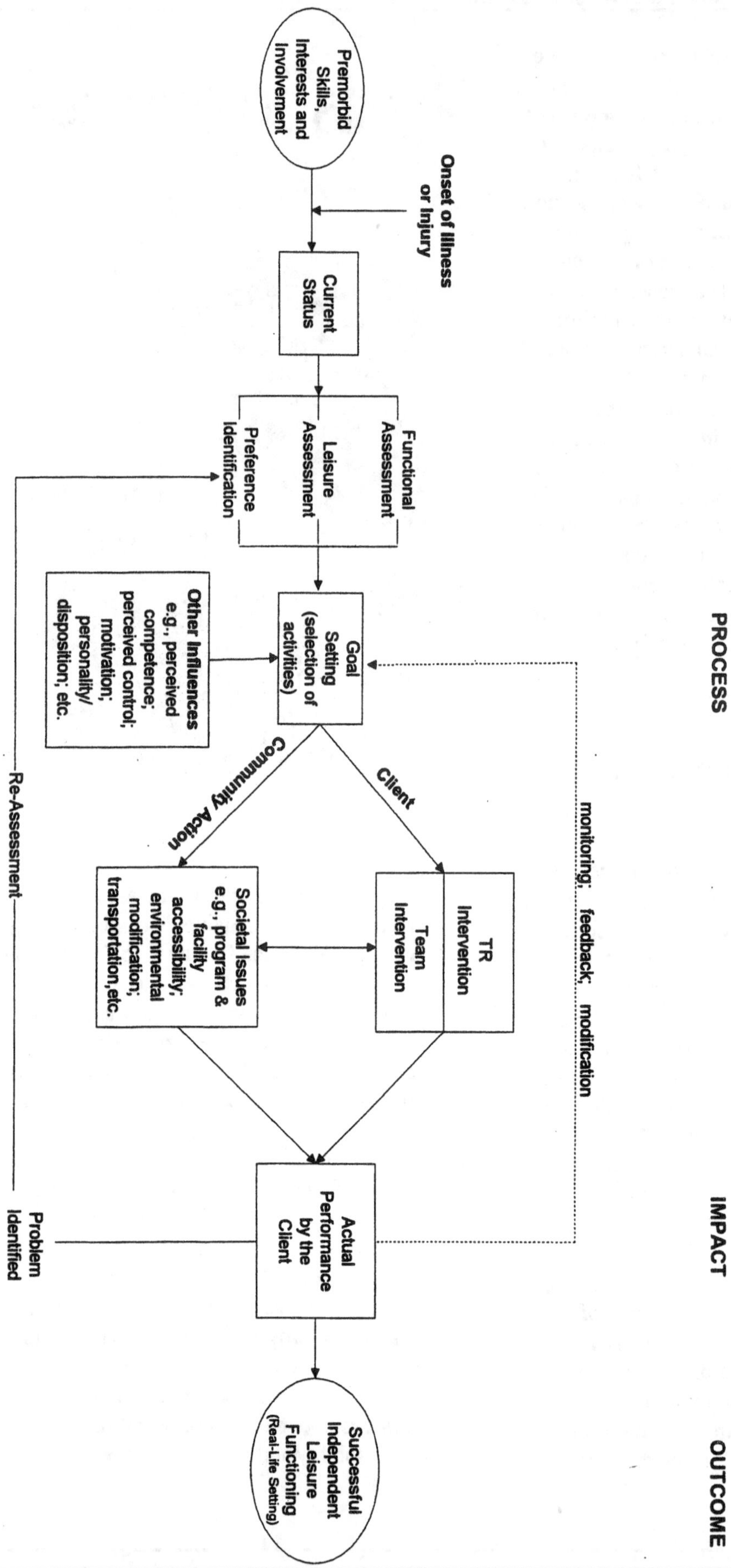

FIGURE 11. THE CLIENT FOCUSED THERAPEUTIC RECREATION PROCESS AND "FIT" OF THE LCM

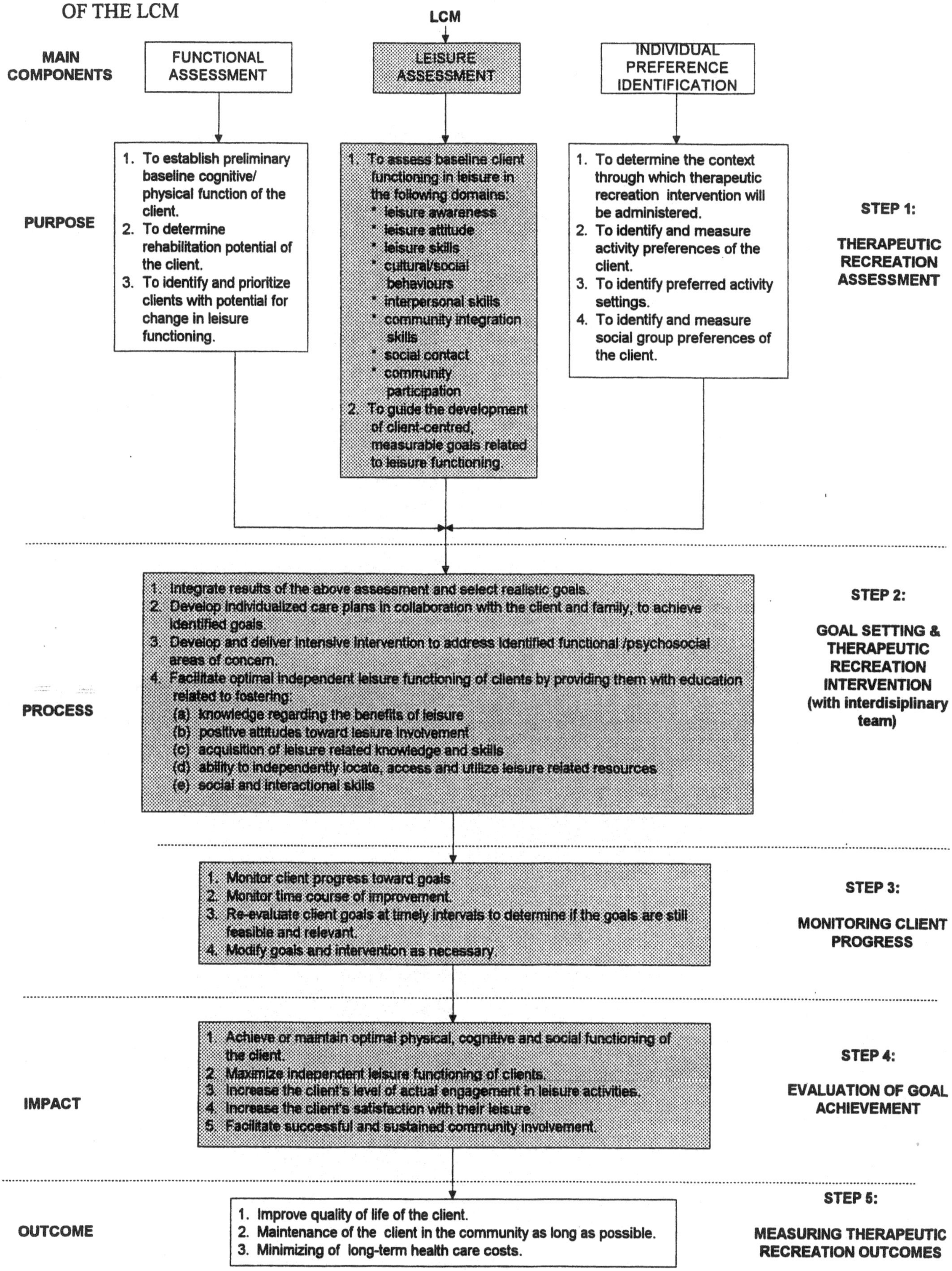

FIGURE 12. THE PROCESS OF THERAPEUTIC PROGRAM FUNCTION AND EVALUATION

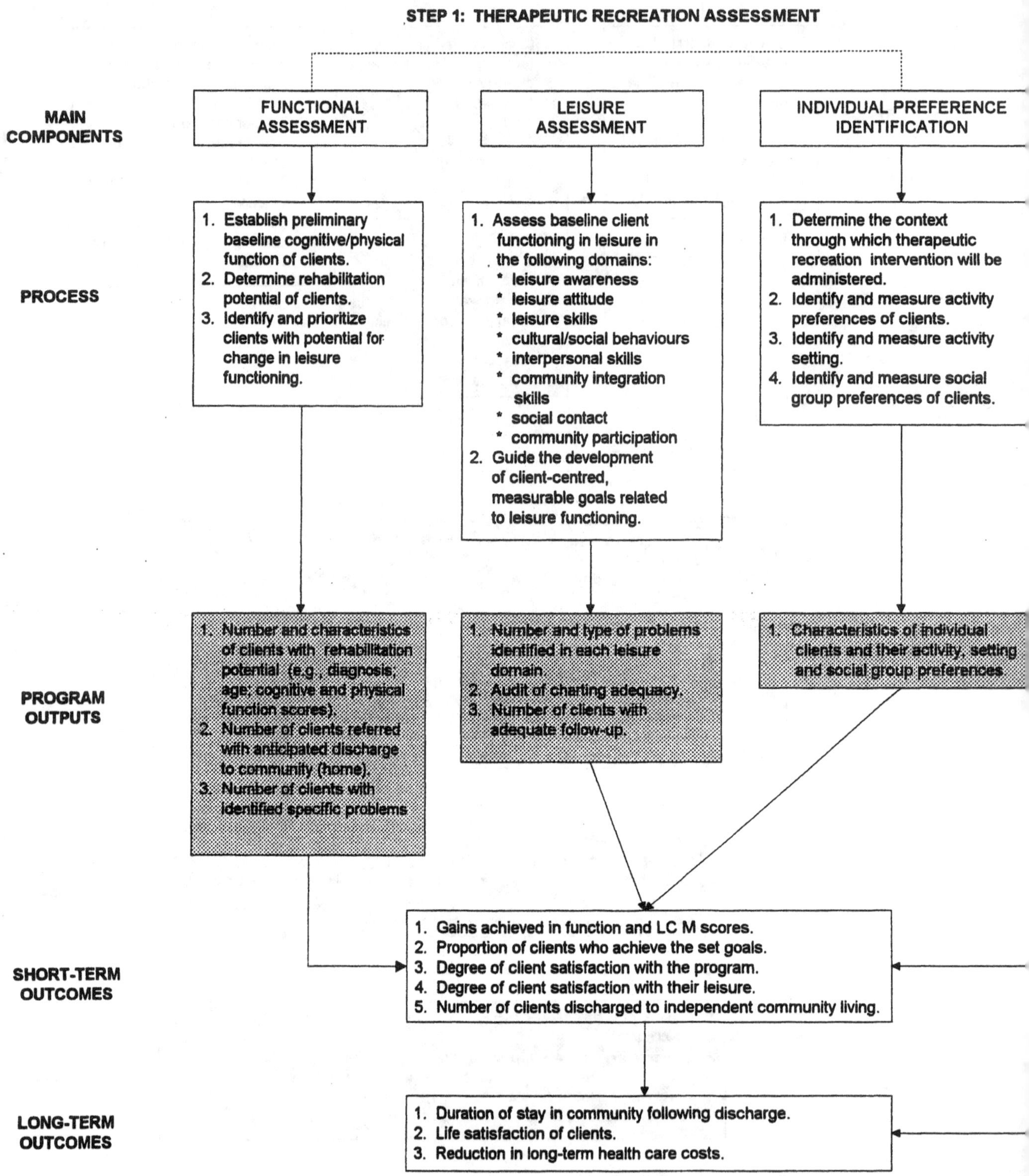

STEP 2

GOAL SETTING AND THERAPEUTIC INTERVENTION

1. Develop individualized care plans in collaboration with the client and family, based upon the results of comprehensive functional and leisure assessments.
2. Develop and deliver intensive intervention to address identified functional/ psychosocial areas of concern based upon the leisure ability continuum.
3. Facilitate optimal independent leisure functioning of clients by providing them with education related to fostering:
   (a) knowledge regarding benefits of leisure
   (b) positive attitudes toward leisure involvement
   (c) acquisition of leisure related knowledge and skills
   (d) ability to independently locate, access and utilize leisure related resources
   (e) social and interactional skills

1. Number & types of clients requiring therapeutic recreation intervention.
2. Number & types of goals set.
3. Types of therapeutic recreation intervention provided.
4. Characteristics of clients who function independently in their leisure.

1. Clients' increased knowledge and understanding of leisure.
2. Clients' increased skill and ability related to leisure functioning.

STEPS 3 & 4

MONITORING CLIENT PROGRESS/ GOAL ACHIEVEMENT EVALUATION

1. Monitor client progress toward goals.
2. Monitor client goals at timely intervals to determine if goals goals are still feasible and relevant.
3. Modify goals and intervention as necessary.
4. Monitor goal achievement at several different times during the program to determine when the most change occurs and when further intervention has minimal effect.

1. Number of goals achieved.
2. Degree of goal achievement.
3. Frequency of goal modification.
4. Hours of therapeutic recreation practitioners' time.
5. Audit of charting adequacy.

STEP 5

FOLLOW-UP DATA COLLECTION

1. Determine carry over of functional gains achieved during intervention, treatment or rehabilitation.
2. Determine clients' actual engagement in leisure activities.
3. Evaluate client satisfaction with leisure.
4. Record and evaluate client functioning in 6-8 weeks post-discharge.

1. Number of clients evaluated and followed-up.
2. Characteristics of clients post-discharge.
3. Number and type of clients routinely engaging in leisure activities.
4. Number and type of clients satisfied with their leisure.
5. Numbers of clients discharged.
6. Types of discharge locations.

Conclusion

We have attempted in this chapter to review some of the potential theoretical bases relevant to therapeutic recreation practice. There are number of defined concepts (constructs) that can contribute to the construction of the overall theoretical framework of the therapeutic recreation profession. We have shown how some of the concepts have been utilized in the construction of the LCM.

It should be clear from the foregoing, how the LCM takes its place in the overall field of therapeutic recreation assessment, goal setting and therapeutic intervention. It is part of an overall picture, all of which is needed for a successful program. We have included in this chapter some simple conceptual models to guide our intervention with clients. Treatment or rehabilitation is a complex, multifaceted activity and we have not intended to oversimplify the process. We hope, however, that these models will help therapeutic professionals in seeing their way through the overall process. A guide, using the Program Logic Model approach illustrates how program activity (outputs) and success of a program can be evaluated. There are many ways of doing this, but a full discussion of program evaluation is beyond the scope of this manual. Nevertheless, we include this example to highlight the importance we attach to this process. Program evaluation references have also been included at the end of this chapter.

References

1. Shank, J.W., Coyle, C.P., Boyd, R. & Kinney, W.B. (1996). A classification scheme for therapeutic recreation research grounded in the rehabilitative sciences. Therapeutic Recreation Journal, 30(3), 179-196.

2. Bedini, L. & Wu, Y. (1994). A methodological review of research in *Therapeutic Recreation Journals* from 1986 to 1990. Therapeutic Recreation Journal, 28(2), 87-98.

3. Stumbo, N.J. (1986). A definition of entry-level knowledge for therapeutic recreation practice. Therapeutic Recreation Journal, 20(4), 15-30.

4. Sylvester, C.D. (1989). Impressions of the intellectual past and future of therapeutic recreation: Implications for professionalism. In D.M. Compton (Ed.), Issues in Therapeutic Recreation: A Profession in Transition (pp. 1-20). Illinois, Sagamore.

5. Ellis, G.D. (1989). The role of science in therapeutic recreation. In D.M. Compton (Ed.), Issues in Therapeutic Recreation: A Profession in Transition (pp. 109-123). Illinois: Sagamore.

6. Mannell, R.C. & Kleiber, D. (1997). A social psychology of leisure. Pennsylvania: Venture.

7. Birren, J.E. & Schaie, K.W. (Eds.) (1985). Handbook of the psychology of aging. New York: Van Nostrand Reinhold.

8. Neulinger, J. (1974). The psychology of leisure. Illinois: Charles C. Thomas.

9. Iso-Ahola, S.E. (1980). Social psychological perspectives on leisure and recreation. Illinois: Charles C. Thomas.

10. Deci, E.L. (1975). Intrinsic motivation. New York: Plenum.

11. Harter, S. (1978). Effectance motivation reconsidered: Toward a developmental model. Human Development. 21, 34-64.

12. Maslow, A.H. (1943). A theory of human motivation. Psychological Review, 50, 370-396.

13. White, R.W. (1959). Motivation reconsidered: The concept of competence. Psychological Review, 66(5), 297-333.

14. Deci, E.L & Ryan, R.M. (1985). Intrinsic motivation and self-determination in human behavior. New York: Plenum.

15. Bandura, A. (1977). Self-efficacy: Toward a unifying theory of behavioral change. Psychological Review, 8, 191-215.

16. Bandura, A. (1986). Social foundations of thought and action: A social cognition theory. New Jersey: Prentice-Hall

17. Rotter, J.B. (1966). Generalized expectancies for internal versus external control of reinforcement. Psychological Monograph: General and Applied, 80, 1-28.

18. Seligman, M.E.P. (1975). Helplessness: On depression, development and death. San Francisco: Freeman.

19. Csikszentimihaly, M. (1990). Flow: The psychology of optimal experience. New York: Harper and Rowe.

20. Ellis, M.J. (1973). Why people play. New Jersey: Prentice-Hall.

21. Lawton, M.P. & Nahemow, L. (1973). Ecology and the aging process. In C. Eisdorfer & M.P. Lawton (Eds.), The Psychology of Adult Development and Aging (pp. 619-674). Washington, D.C.: American Psychological Association.

22. Kahana, E. (1982). A congruence model of person-environment interaction. In M.P. Lawton, P.G. Windley, & T.O. Byerts (Eds.), Aging and the Environment: Theoretical Approaches (pp. 97-121). New York: Springer.

23. Lazarus, R.S. & Folkman, S. (1984). Stress, appraisal and coping. New York: Springer.

24. Pastalam, L.A. (1982). Research in environmental aging: An alternative to theory. In M.P. Lawton, P.G. Windley & T. O. Byerts (Eds.), Aging and the Environment: Theoretical Approaches (pp. 122-131). New York: Springer.

25. Havighurst, R.J. & Albrecht, R. (1953). Older people. New York: Longmans, Green and Co.

26. Atchley, R. (1988). A continuity theory of normal aging. The Gerontologist, 29, 183-190.

27. Fuhrer, M.J. (1987). Overview of outcome analysis in rehabilitation. In M.J. Fuhrer (Ed.), Rehabilitation Outcomes: Analysis and Measurement (pp. 1-15). Baltimore: Paul H. Brookes.

28. World Health Organization (1980). International classification of impairments, disability, and handicaps: A manual of classification relating to the consequences of disease. Geneva: Author.

29. Peterson, C.A. & Gunn, S. (1984). Therapeutic recreation program design: Principles and procedures (2nd Ed.). New Jersey: Prentice-Hall.

30. Ford, M.E. (1985). The concept of competence: Themes and variations. In H.A. Marlowe Jr. & R.B. Weinberg (Eds.), Competence Development: Theory and Practice in Special Populations (pp. 3-49). Illinois: Charles C. Thomas.

31. Gerard, R. (1959). Aging and levels of organization. In J. Birren (Ed.), Handbook of Aging and the Individual (pp. 264-273). Chicago: University of Chicago Press.

32. Hogg, J.R. & Hillary, K. (1990). A measure of relational competence for community-dwelling elderly. Psychology and Aging, 5(4), 580-588.

33. Lawton, M.P. (1972). Assessing the competence of older people. In D.P. Kent, R. Kastenbaum & S. Sherwood (Eds.), Research, Planning and Action for the Elderly: The Power and Potential of Social Science (pp. 122-143). New York: John Wiley.

34. Norris, N. (1991). The trouble with competence. Cambridge Journal of Education, 21(3), 331-341.

35. Kloseck, M., Crilly, R.G., Ellis, G.D. & Lammers, E. (1996). Leisure Competence Measure: Development and reliability of a scale to measure functional outcomes in therapeutic recreation. Therapeutic Recreation Journal, 30(1), 13-26.

36. Kemp, B., Brummel-Smith, K. & Ramsdell, J.W. (1990). Geriatric Rehabilitation. Boston: College-Hill.

37. Wagner, K.A. (1987). Outcome analysis in comprehensive medical rehabilitation. In M.J. Fuhrer (Ed.), Rehabilitation Outcomes: Analysis and Measurement (pp. 19-28). Baltimore: Paul H. Brookes.

38. Nagi, S.Z. (1976). An epidemiology of disability among adults in the United States. Health and Society, 439-467.

39. Nagi, S. (1991). Disability concepts revisited: Implications for prevention. In A.M. Pope & A.R. Tarlov (Eds.), Disability in America: Toward a National Agenda for Prevention (pp. 309-327). Washington, D.C.: National Academy Press.

40. Pope, A.M. & Tarlov, A.R. (Eds.) (1991) Disability in America: Toward a National Agenda for Prevention. Washington, D.C.: National Academy Press.

41. Hamilton, B.B., Granger, F.S., Zielezny, M. & Tashman, J.S. (1987). A uniform national data system for medical rehabilitation. In M.J. Fuhrer (Ed.), Rehabilitation Outcomes: Analysis and Measurement (pp. 137-147). Baltimore: Paul H. Brookes.

42. Johnston, M.V., Keith, R.A. & Hinderer, S.R. (1992). Measurement standards for interdisciplinary medical rehabilitation. Archives of Physical Medicine and Rehabilitation, 73, S-3-S-23.

43. Studenski, S. & Duncan, P.W. (1993). Measuring rehabilitation outcomes. Clinics in Geriatric Medicine, 9(4), 823-830.

44. Baltes, M.M., Mayr, U., Borchelt, M., Maas, I. & Wilms, H.U. (1993). Everyday competence in old and very old age: An inter-disciplinary perspective. Aging and Society, 13, 657-680.

45. Baltes, M. M. (1988). Etiology and maintenance of dependency in the elderly: Three phases of operant research. Behavior Therapy, 19, 301-319.

46. Baltes, M.M. & Wahl, H.W. (1992). The behavior system of dependency in the elderly: Interaction with the social environment. In M.G. Ory, R.P. Abeles & P.D. Lipman (Eds.), Aging, Health and Behavior (pp. 83-106). Newbury Park, California: Sage.

47. Mundy, J. & Odum, L. (1979). Leisure education: Theory and practice. New York: John Wiley.

48. Riddick, C.C. (1986). Leisure satisfaction precursors. Journal of Leisure Research, 18(4), 259-265.

49. Searle, M.S. & Mahon, M.J. (1991). Leisure education in a day hospital: The effects on selected social-psychological variables among older adults. Canadian Journal of Community Mental Health, 10(2), 95-109.

50. Searle, M.S. & Mahon, M.J. (1993). The effects of a leisure education program on selected social-psychological variables: A three month follow-up investigation. Therapeutic Recreation Journal, 27(1), 9-21.

51. Searle, M.S., Mahon, M.J., Iso-Ahola, S.E., Sdrolias, H.A. & Van Dyck, J. (1995). Enhancing a sense of independence and psychological well-being among the elderly: A field experiment. Journal of Leisure Research, 27(2), 107-124.

52. Bloom, M., Fischer, J. & Orme, J.G. (1995). Evaluating practice: Guidelines for the accountable professional. London: Allyn and Bacon.

53. Rossi, P.H. & Freeman, H.E. (1993). Evaluation: A systematic approach. Newbury Park, California: Sage.

54. Mohr, L.B. (1992). Impact analysis for program evaluation. Newbury Park, California: Sage.

55. Hudson, J., Mayne, J. & Thomlison, R. (1992). Action-oriented evaluation in organizations: Canadian practices. Toronto, Ontario: Wall and Emerson, Inc.

56. Fink, A. (1993). Evaluation fundamentals: Guiding health programs, research and policy. Newbury Park, California: Sage.

CHAPTER 3

Leisure Competence Measure

SUMMARY

- *The LCM is not an assessment tool, rather a way to summarize and categorize information gathered from a variety of sources as part of the therapeutic recreation assessment process.*

- *The LCM consists of 8 subscales. The first 6 subscales measure client capabilities; the remaining 2 subscales measure actual performance of the client.*

- *The LCM is scored on a 7-level hierarchical scale (7 = complete independence; 1 = total dependence) and is consistent with the FIM.*

- *The LCM may be used either for screening purposes, or for full evaluation of a client's functioning in leisure; subscales may be scored separately or scores may be summed to produce a total leisure functioning score.*

- *The LCM has been tested in a variety of settings including geriatric, rehabilitation and psychiatric settings, and with clients with a wide range of diagnoses.*

- *Once learned, average time to complete LCM ratings per client (once the therapeutic recreation assessment has been completed) is 5 minutes or less.*

- *Results of testing to date support the LCM as an instrument from which valid and dependable inferences regarding leisure functioning may be drawn for clients in general and specialized rehabilitation settings, as well as geriatric settings.*

- *It is the responsibility of all test users to understand the psychometric properties of the instruments they are using.*

Chapter 3
Administering, Scoring and Interpreting the LCM

Introduction

The LCM provides one means of beginning to standardize and ensure uniformity in assessment procedures, goal setting and the delivery of therapeutic recreation intervention. The LCM provides the profession with a core set of leisure functioning measures, consistently defined and uniformly applied, with information related to leisure functioning that all therapeutic recreation professionals interpret in a similar way. This will allow practitioners and researchers to more accurately compare therapeutic recreation intervention and program results among similar facilities and similar client populations. It is also a scale that is easily recognized by other health professionals and agencies who are familiar with the Functional Independence Measure (FIM). The LCM was designed to be consistent with the FIM, an outcome measure for rehabilitation and is therefore ideal for goal setting and evaluation in an inter-disciplinary team setting. Establishment of a computerized data base of LCM change scores could potentially provide practitioners, agencies and the profession with normative data and comparisons of client scores on a regional, national and international level. The LCM international comparative data base has the potential of becoming a valuable data base for ongoing research supporting the efficacy of therapeutic recreation.

The LCM serves as a standard means of categorizing and summarizing information related to leisure functioning. It is an instrument that has been rigorously tested, over time and demonstrates evidence of good validity and reliability. The LCM is simple, easily built into daily practice and useful across a variety of disabilities and settings. Evaluation of LCM change scores, examination of intervention effectiveness and the development of normative data will enable more accurate identification of the role of therapeutic recreation in the health care delivery system.

Purpose of the LCM

One of the primary goals of therapeutic recreation intervention is to assist individuals in developing specific skills, knowledge and behaviours that will allow them to function independently, enjoy their leisure optimally and, where appropriate, live successfully and independently in the community with the least amount of assistance possible. Outcome measures, then, are necessary to record how fully these goals are achieved.

The LCM provides therapeutic recreation practitioners with a tool to document change in leisure functioning. The LCM provides a means of identifying initial levels of individual functioning in eight leisure domains identified as necessary indicators of competence in leisure. These domains include leisure awareness, leisure attitude, leisure skills, cultural/social behaviours, interpersonal skills, community integration, social contact and community participation. The first six subscales measure "readiness for" successful and independent functioning in leisure. The remaining two subscales measure actual client engagement or performance. The components of the LCM were summarized in Table 4 (pg. 33), which for ease of reference is reproduced here as Table 5.

TABLE 5. COMPONENTS OF THE LEISURE COMPETENCE MEASURE (Table 4 reproduced for ease of reference)

LCM SUBSCALES	DESCRIPTION	TYPE OF MEASUREMENT
Leisure Awareness	Client's knowledge and understanding of leisure.	MEASURE OF CLIENT CAPABILITIES
Leisure Attitude	Behaviours exhibited and/or feelings demonstrated by the client which suggest attitude toward leisure involvement.	
Leisure Skills	Skills possessed by the client which affect leisure involvement.	
Cultural/Social Behaviours	Specific cultural/social behaviours exhibited by the client which affect his/her ability to function effectively in leisure activities.	
Interpersonal Skills	Client's ability to participate within various types of inter-individual and/or group situations.	
Community Integration Skills	Application of antecedent skills for successful involvement in community leisure activities.	
Social Contact	Type and duration of social contact the client has with others.	MEASURE OF CLIENT ACTUAL PERFORMANCE
Community Participation	Client's overall leisure participation pattern within the community.	

The LCM was also designed to:

- ❑ determine a client's current level of leisure functioning
- ❑ assist therapeutic recreation professionals in establishing specific goals for their clients
- ❑ monitor individual client progress (change in function) over time
- ❑ evaluate the effectiveness of therapeutic recreation intervention
- ❑ better predict potential of clients with varying diagnoses
- ❑ classify leisure functioning for future research purposes

The LCM is not an assessment tool and is not intended to replace existing therapeutic recreation assessment tools. Rather, the LCM is a summarization of the assessment process and should be used to summarize and categorize information related to overall client functioning, gathered through a variety of sources (e.g., client assessment; client observation; interview with client's family; the client's medical record; team discussion; etc). Upon completion of the initial therapeutic recreation assessment (e.g., collecting information regarding general functioning, leisure functioning and interests), the LCM requires that skills and/or behaviours be evaluated, in each of the eight domains, by seven functional levels, ranging from complete independence to total dependence (see Tables 6 and 7). Goals are set and progress is evaluated on the 7-level scale (7=complete independence; 1=total dependence). Rankings of 5 or below represent varying degrees of dependent functioning, and rankings of 6 and 7 represent degrees of independent functioning. These levels of functioning are consistent throughout all LCM subscales (Tables 6 and 7). The focus is on the ***behaviour*** of the client, ***not*** the activity the client is involved in. By isolating behaviours impacting on leisure functioning it becomes possible to assign a numerical value to leisure functioning. These values are recorded using the LCM data sheet (Figure 28, p.84). To achieve a score of 7 the client must be able to function independently with *no* verbal or physical intervention *at all.* Adaptive devices are ***not*** considered a form of dependency if they are utilized independently.

<u>Important Note</u>:

The LCM subscales are intended to measure what the client ***actually does***, not what he/she ***ought*** to be able to do.

Intervention strategies can then be developed consistent with identified levels of functioning on each scale. Intervention priorities should be with those domains having the ***greatest negative impact*** on ***immediate*** client functioning, then proceed to those domains having a lesser impact. For example, when working with a client scoring low on the social contact, interpersonal skills and leisure skills scales (e.g., social contact = 3; interpersonal skills =3; leisure skills =4), it is more important to work with the client on developing and supporting specific interpersonal skills in order that the client may more successfully participate in group situations ***before*** setting social contact goals which require these interpersonal skills to be intact for successful and sustained contact with the client's family, friends and

"...fun is the steadfast goal of recreation, but not its purpose."
Paul Haun

"... the individuals most in need of recreation involvement are least able to obtain it voluntarily."
Dr. Fred Humphrey

community in general. Client progress is then monitored and documented, over time, and a final rating is assigned to LCM subscales at the time of the client's discharge. This allows identification and measurement of change in client leisure functioning (outcomes derived from defined therapeutic recreation intervention) in leisure between admission and discharge (Figures 13 to 18).

TABLE 6. LCM FUNCTIONAL LEVELS

LEVELS	7 Complete Independence 6 Modified Independence	**NO HELPER**
	5 Modified Dependence 4 Modified Dependence with Minimal Assistance 3 Modified Dependence with Moderate Assistance 2 Modified Dependence with Maximal Assistance 1 Total Dependence with Total Assistance	**HELPER**

Important Note:

Clients must meet *all* the requirements within a given functional level. If the client does not meet *all* requirements, he or she must automatically fall to the level below, and be assigned the ranking of that lower category.

The LCM is useful as a goal setting and program planning tool. Competencies identified through the LCM can be used to encourage the client to work on improving or developing behaviours necessary for more independent functioning in their leisure. Progress in developing competencies can be documented through increased levels of ability as recorded on the LCM data sheet. Programs can be modified as needed to meet the changing needs of individual clients. The LCM is designed to be used for screening (to objectively determine those individuals who are a priority for therapeutic recreation intervention) and full assessment purposes (see Figure 29, pg. 86). The last two subscales of the LCM (social contact and community participation) are designed to be discipline independent and may be utilized by other health professionals (e.g., nursing; home care workers; physiotherapists; occupational therapists; etc.) to identify clients at risk. This approach will allow for earlier intervention and perhaps delay institutionalization by providing support through existing community-based recreation programs. The LCM was designed for both therapeutic recreation practice and research purposes. LCM indicators are useful for program evaluation and goal achievement analysis as part of continuous quality improvement procedures and an international data base is being established for research purposes.

Population

The LCM was originally designed for use in adult rehabilitation, geriatric, psychiatric and long-term care settings and has also been found useful by practitioners working with young adults and adolescents (13+ years). The leisure education principles upon which

TABLE 7. TYPE OF INTERVENTION REQUIRED FOR LCM FUNCTIONAL LEVELS

Functional Level	Type of Intervention Required
7 6	no intervention
5	verbal cueing
4 3 2 1	physical assistance

the LCM depends, while applicable to adults, are not applicable to children. A different conceptual basis, notably theories of play and developmental theories, will form the basis of the paediatric version of the LCM which is currently under development (expected 1998).

Testing, to date, of the adult version has been conducted in rehabilitation settings (e.g., spinal cord injury; brain injury; general neurological conditions; multi-trauma; stroke; etc.) and with a geriatric rehabilitation population. In the pilot study (see pg. 59) it was suggested that the LCM would also be valuable for psychiatric settings. While therapeutic recreation practitioners working in psychiatric settings are using the LCM and have confirmed that they find this tool helpful, full testing with this population remains to be done.

Severity and Condition of Clients with Whom the LCM was Tested

In rehabilitation, the LCM has been tested with clients who have sustained acute injuries (traumatic recent injury) with a Glasgow Coma Scale score of 9 or more and Rancho Scale score of IV or higher. Ventilator dependent clients were not included in LCM testing. The geriatric population with whom the LCM has been tested were clients, with a Mini-Mental State Examination (MMSE) score ≥ 23; clients with scores < 23 were not included in the validation of the LCM.

Logically it would appear unreasonable to apply the leisure education model to cognitively impaired clients, where learning is unlikely to occur and confusion is increasing. In practice, however, therapeutic recreation professionals have used the LCM with clients in special care units and Alzheimer units[1] and reported it valuable, in the absence of other available standardized measures specific to therapeutic recreation for this population. Therapeutic recreation professionals on these units have not monitored progress over time, rather behavioural and functional *decline*. This approach has helped to more objectively determine when clients should be moved from higher to lower functioning programs due, for example, to increasingly disruptive behaviour. Changes inconsistent with cognitive ability may also highlight the need for intervention. The aim of therapeutic recreation professionals in Alzheimer units and special care units is to ensure that their clients function at their optimal level of *limited* functioning, for as long as possible.

Settings

The LCM has been used and tested in a variety of settings. Settings within which the LCM has been tested include general and special rehabilitation units, geriatric rehabilitation units and geriatric day hospital settings. The LCM is also being widely used in psychiatric and community settings, as well as with physically disabled adolescents in both in-patient and outpatient settings. Validity and reliability testing in these settings and with these populations is currently underway.

Much more rigorous testing of the LCM is necessary to fully evaluate the LCM's usefulness across a variety of settings, including some of the above. It is our hope that the international comparative data base will, in time, perform this function.

Time to Complete the LCM

Although the LCM may look lengthy, therapeutic recreation professionals using the LCM report that, once learned, it is actually very quick and easy to complete. Studies show that the initial time to *learn* to use the LCM is for the vast majority of practitioners under 1 hour. Once the therapeutic recreation assessment has been completed, average time per client to complete the LCM is initially around 10 minutes. With practice, the time per client to complete the LCM has been reported as 5 minutes or less.

Cost and Material Required

Other than the LCM (8 subscales) and the LCM data sheet, no additional material or cost is required. The major cost is in practitioner time, which studies have shown is minimal. Windows-based LCM software, designed to assist practitioners and agencies in collecting and summarizing large amounts of data, is optional. This software was designed to quickly and easily transform numerical LCM data into high impact visual format that may then be incorporated into other programs (e.g., WordPerfect) for quarterly continuous quality improvement reports, reports for payers/purchasers of therapeutic recreation services, administrators and others.

Training Required

The 2 subscales of the LCM that measure actual engagement and social contact abilities of the client (social contact and community participation) are designed to be discipline independent and may be used by any allied health professionals (e.g., nurses; social workers; home care physiotherapists and occupational therapists; etc.) to identify clients at risk. The remaining 6 subscales which target specific problem areas are specific to the therapeutic recreation discipline and require professional knowledge and training that typifies the field. These 6 LCM subscales are operationalized through leisure education principles and measure client capabilities related specifically to leisure functioning (e.g., leisure awareness; leisure attitude; leisure skills; cultural/social behaviours; interpersonal skills; community integration). Studies and training session results have demonstrated that professionals with the designation Certified Therapeutic Recreation Specialist (CTRS) who are certified through the National Council for Therapeutic Recreation Certification (NCTRC), and those professionals with formal education in therapeutic recreation and leisure education principles, produced more accurate, consistent and reliable scores on the LCM subscales. Special training is required in therapeutic recreation assessment procedures and leisure education models in order to ensure that the 6 LCM subscales measuring client capabilities related to leisure functioning are used correctly.

Training in the use of the LCM will allow therapeutic recreation professionals to turn the results of their assessments into a score on the LCM. However, the LCM score will only be as good as the therapeutic recreation assessment and the understanding of the leisure education principles upon which the

LCM is constructed. This in turn is dependent upon the knowledge, training and skills of the therapeutic recreation professional in this area.

For research purposes, the LCM has been shown to be reliable and sensitive to change. However, conducting research implies an understanding of research methodology, standardized instruments and intervention so that ultimately valid conclusions may be drawn that link clearly defined therapeutic recreation intervention to outcomes.

Responsibilities of Users of Tests and Instruments

It is important that test users understand: (1) the psychometric properties of the instruments they plan to use; (2) the

TABLE 8. STRENGTHS AND LIMITATIONS OF THE LCM

STRENGTHS	LIMITATIONS
The LCM . . .	The LCM . . .
✔ is a standardized instrument ✔ has evidence of good validity and reliability ✔ has theoretical underpinnings ✔ guides TR intervention ✔ measures outcomes of TR intervention ✔ is useful across a variety of settings and with a variety of client populations ✔ is quick and easy to learn and use ✔ is easily incorporated into every day TR practice ✔ is consistent with the FIM and easily understood by other allied health professionals familiar with the FIM ✔ is consistent with accreditation standards required by such organizations as CARF, JCAHO, and CCHSA ✔ provides valuable information for reports required for continuous quality improvement, payers and purchasers of TR services, administrators, etc. ✔ will provide agencies with their own TR research base ✔ will ultimately provide an international research base for TR	☞ requires TR professionals to have knowledge of specific approaches (e.g., TR assessment procedures; leisure education principles; etc.) ☞ allows comparison of outcomes across agencies, but this implies comparable skills in assessment, goal setting, intervention planning, etc. ☞ cannot make a "bad" assessment "good"

theoretical and conceptual bases of the instrument; (3) for whom the instrument is intended; (4) for which settings the instrument is intended; (5) how to administer, score and interpret instrument results; and (6) any limitations or cautions identified related to the use of the instrument. It is also the responsibility of instrument users to have knowledge related to the domains the instrument measures. Instrument users who modify instruments or deviate from reported administration procedures for the instrument should not use published data describing the psychometric properties of the instrument to support or justify their use of the instrument. Readers wishing more detailed information on general standards for users of measures should refer to the work of Johnston, Keith and Hinderer.[2]

Strengths and Limitations of the LCM

It is important for therapeutic recreation professionals to understand the strengths and weaknesses of the LCM so they can evaluate the appropriateness of the LCM's use in various settings and for various purposes. Table 8 highlights strengths and limitations of the LCM identified through research, training sessions and discussion with therapeutic recreation professionals routinely using the LCM.

Results of testing to date support the LCM as an instrument from which valid and dependable inferences regarding leisure functioning may be drawn for clients in general and specialized rehabilitation settings, as well as geriatric settings. Therapeutic recreation practitioners working in other settings (e.g., psychiatric; adolescent; etc.) have reported that the LCM is also useful and valuable, however detailed testing remains to be carried out in these settings. One of the greatest strengths of the LCM, as reported by practitioners, is that it offers a relatively simple approach to therapeutic recreation outcome evaluation and research that can easily be incorporated into daily practice. This approach allows therapeutic recreation professionals to evaluate changes over time in a single client, as well as compare changes in the outcomes of many clients, across a variety of settings. Examination of intervention effectiveness, evaluation of goal achievement and gain scores, and the development of normative data will enable more accurate identification of the role of therapeutic recreation in the delivery of health services.

Testing the LCM (Does it Work?)

The LCM was developed in 1988 using an iterative process consisting of four phases (pilot, trial, implementation and revision). In 1989 a multi-centre pilot study was conducted to test face validity, reliability and feasibility of the LCM in Canada and the United States[3] and used to make modifications to the LCM. The pilot testing was designed to be consistent with that of the Functional Independence Measure (FIM). Data was collected from rehabilitation, geriatric and psychiatric clients in seven hospitals throughout Canada and the United States and feedback was provided by 25 experts in the field. The jury of experts consisted of 5 therapeutic recreation educators, 18 therapeutic recreation practitioners (average number of years of therapeutic recreation experience = 6) and 2 physicians. Suggestions received from the jury of experts were incorporated into the most recent version of the LCM. During the trial phase and as a preliminary to the implementation phase, more extensive validity and reliability testing, under a variety of possible scenarios, was conducted.[3,4,5,6,7] The following section highlights research studies, carried out to date, utilizing the LCM.

As part of the pilot testing, the expert jury

responded to several questions regarding the LCM:

① Is the LCM an adequate measure of leisure competence? On a scale of 1 (poor) to 5 (excellent) the LCM received an overall rating of 4.0.

② Are any LCM items difficult to understand? Sixty-seven percent reported that all items were easy to understand.

③ Are there any unnecessary items included in the LCM? Seventy-five percent reported all items were necessary.

④ Are there items that should be added to the LCM? One hundred percent said "no".

⑤ The jury of experts was also asked how useful they considered the LCM for use in their facility. On a scale of 1 (poor) to 5 (excellent) the jury rated the usefulness of the LCM as a 4.5.

These questions help to begin to establish content validity. More detailed information on the pilot testing of the LCM may be found in the paper by Kloseck, Crilly, Ellis and Lammers.[3]

Initial testing with a geriatric population (n=52) confirmed the high internal reliability of the LCM as measured by Cronbach's Alpha Reliability Coefficient (α = .97)[6], indicating that the various LCM subscales reflect aspects of a single construct. The high internal consistency of the LCM was further demonstrated in a study (n=114) that examined the LCM employing both classical test theory analysis and generalizability analysis.[3] Classical test theory results produced an α = .92. The dependability component of the generalizability analysis indicated that dependable measures can be obtained by one rater for both the screening subscales (Social Contact and Community Participation) and the LCM as a whole. G coefficients of greater than .89 were found for the total LCM and subscales for the worst case scenario (only one rater) indicating high internal consistency of the total LCM scale and subscales. This supports both uses of the scale, for screening and full evaluation purposes, and the adequacy of a single rater scoring the LCM, important considerations for its application in daily therapeutic recreation practice.

Initial studies also demonstrated significant correlations between scores on the LCM and measures of other phenomena which would be expected to impact leisure competence.[5,6,7] For example, statistically significant correlations were found with: (1) measures of confusion, assessed by the Mini-Mental State Examination (MMSE);[15] (2) depression as measured by the Geriatric Depression Scale (GDS);[16] and (3) life satisfaction as measured by the Life Satisfaction Index (LSIB).[17] These demonstrated correlations lend support to criterion-related validity of the LCM. A sample of 47 subjects was used to assess inter-rater reliability. The Intra-Class Correlation was quite satisfactory for the total LCM scale (r = .91).

A follow-up study (n=107), using a path analytic approach, examined the LCM as a predictor variable in building an exploratory model of the determinants of life satisfaction in a geriatric rehabilitation population.[5] Leisure and functional skills leading to active community participation and social contact were hypothesized as an appropriate pathway to life satisfaction. Path analytic results of this study, using LISREL, supported the community participation to social contact to life satisfaction path and also, as predicted, supported the significant contribution of leisure attitude, leisure skills and physical function to community participation and group interaction skills on social contact. Surprisingly leisure awareness and depression contributed little to the model. The proportion of the variance of life satisfaction explained by the model is 34%.

This successful involvement of the LCM in

initial (exploratory) model building among a variety of other measures reinforces the LCM as an independent phenomenon and lends support to the LCM's construct validity.

In a recent retrospective study (n=640)[4] which examined LCM admission and discharge scores from consecutive admissions to geriatric and rehabilitation units in two major hospitals in Canada (over a 2 year period) and the United States (over a 4 year period), the LCM was shown to be sensitive to change over time in geriatric, as well as general and specialized rehabilitation settings (see Figures 13-18), supporting the LCM's value as a measure sufficiently sensitive to reflect client outcomes. Likewise, the LCM was sensitive to diagnostic category (Figure 19). Internal reliability of the LCM in this study, as measured by Cronbach's Alpha Reliability Coefficient, was again quite satisfactory (∝ = .93).

Results of these preliminary studies examining the LCM, support that valid and dependable inferences may be made regarding leisure functioning of clients with a variety of diagnoses, across a variety of settings.

FIGURE 13. EXAMPLE 1: ACTUAL LCM SCORES FOR A CLIENT ADMITTED TO A GERIATRIC DAY HOSPITAL

72 year old male diagnosed as having a stroke. Length of stay in the day hospital was approximately 6 months.

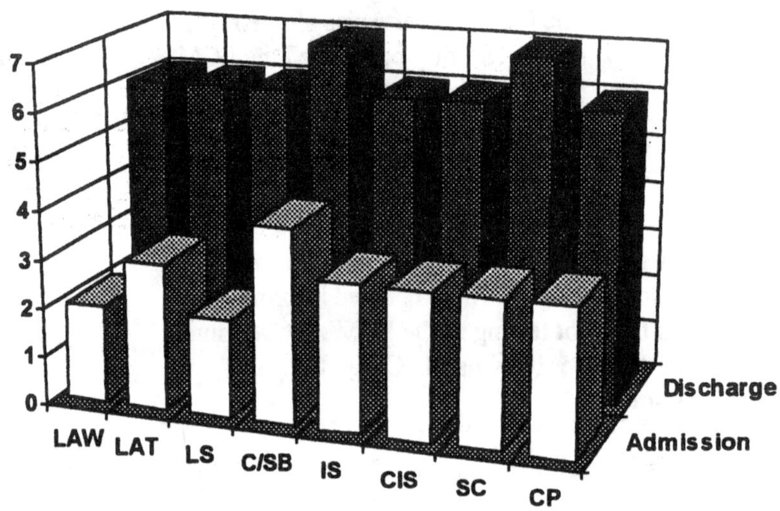

Legend:

LAW = Leisure Awareness
LAT = Leisure Attitude
LS = Leisure Skills
C/SB = Cultural/Social Behaviours
IS = Interpersonal Skills
CIS = Community Integration Skills
SC = Social Contact
CP = Community Participation

FIGURE 14. EXAMPLE 2: ACTUAL LCM SCORES FOR A CLIENT ADMITTED TO A GERIATRIC DAY HOSPITAL

76 year old male diagnosed with Parkinson's disease. Length of stay in the day hospital was approximately 5 months.

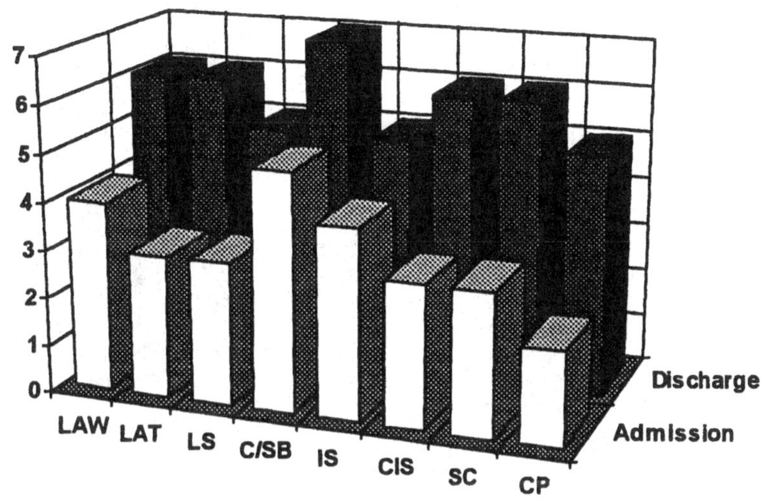

FIGURE 15. EXAMPLE 3: ACTUAL LCM SCORES FOR A CLIENT ADMITTED TO A BRAIN INJURY UNIT

59 year old female diagnosed with a traumatic brain injury due to a fall down a flight of stairs. Length of stay in the unit was approximately 2 months prior to discharge home.

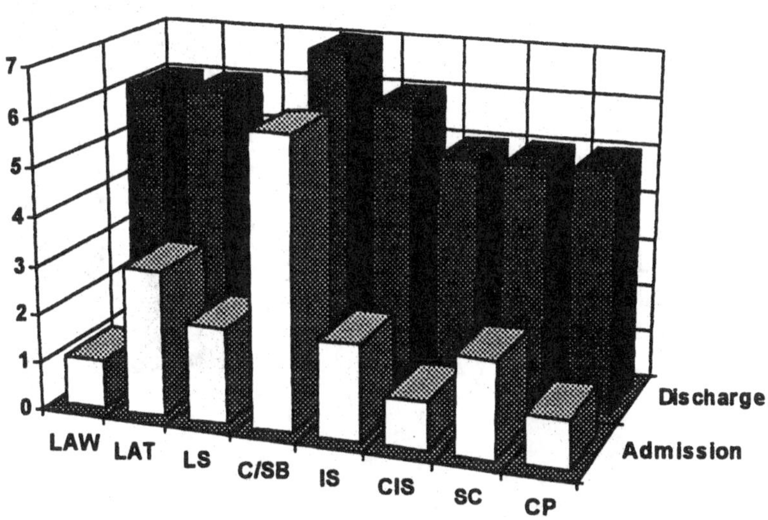

FIGURE 16. EXAMPLE 4: ACTUAL LCM SCORES FOR A CLIENT ADMITTED TO A BRAIN INJURY UNIT

42 year old male diagnosed with a traumatic brain injury due to a motorcycle accident. Length of stay in the unit was approximately 3 months.

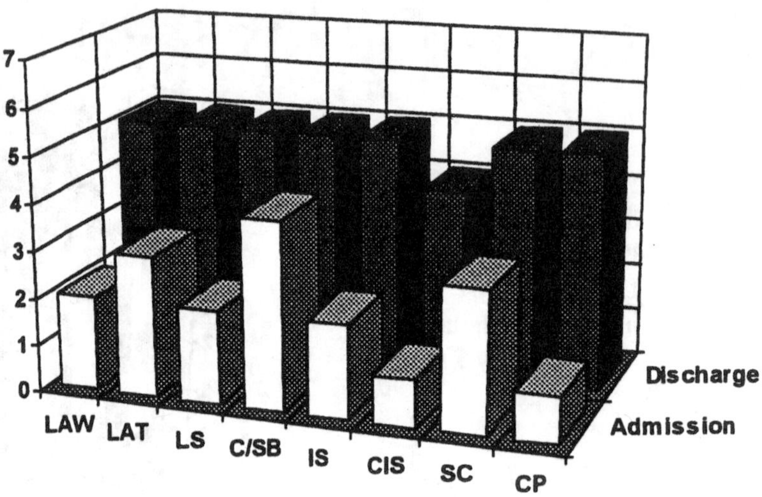

FIGURE 17. EXAMPLE 5: ACTUAL LCM SCORES FOR A CLIENT ADMITTED TO A SPINAL CORD INJURY UNIT

19 year old female diagnosed with a spinal cord injury due to a boating accident. Length of stay in the unit was approximately 4 months.

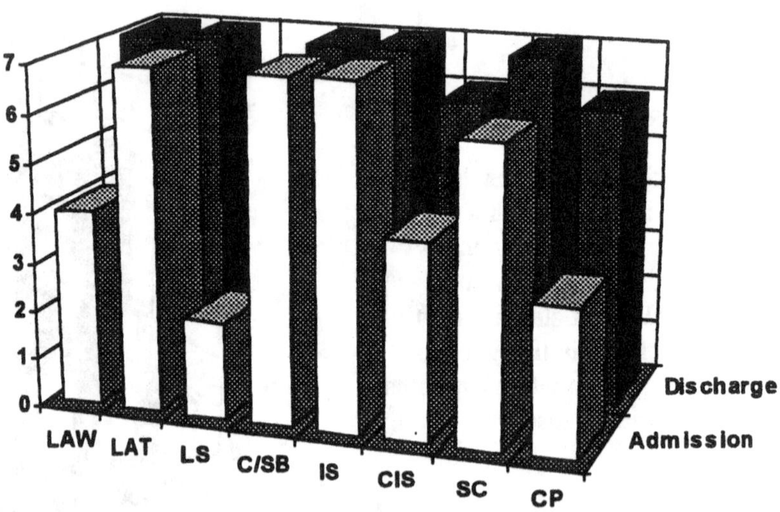

FIGURE 18. EXAMPLE 6: ACTUAL LCM SCORES FOR A CLIENT ADMITTED TO A SPINAL CORD INJURY UNIT

21 year old male diagnosed with a spinal cord injury due to a motor vehicle accident. Length of stay in the unit was approximately 2 months.

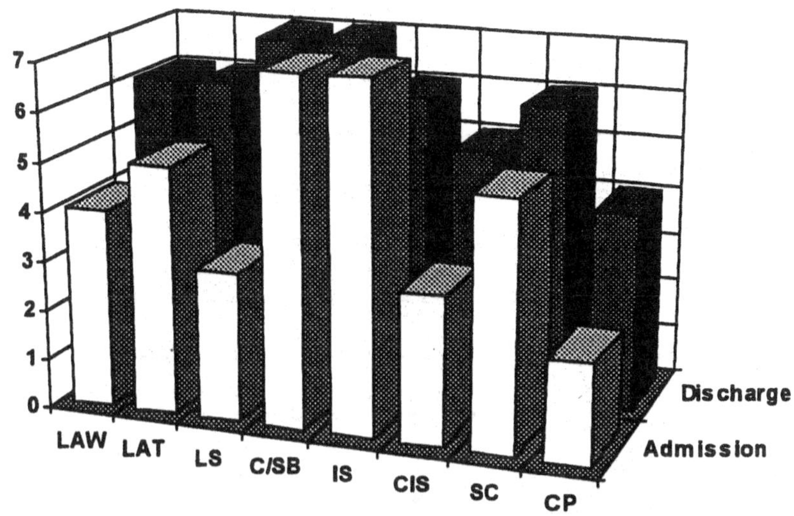

Legend:

LAW	= Leisure Awareness
LAT	= Leisure Attitude
LS	= Leisure Skills
C/SB	= Cultural/Social Behaviours
IS	= Interpersonal Skills
CIS	= Community Integration Skills
SC	= Social Contact
CP	= Community Participation

FIGURE 19. PROFILES OF MEAN LCM ADMISSION AND DISCHARGE SCORES BY DIAGNOSTIC CATEGORY

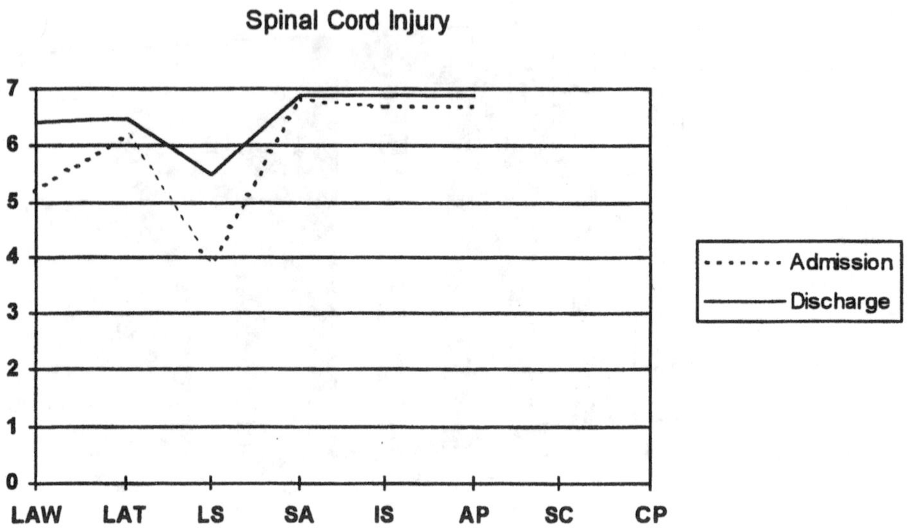

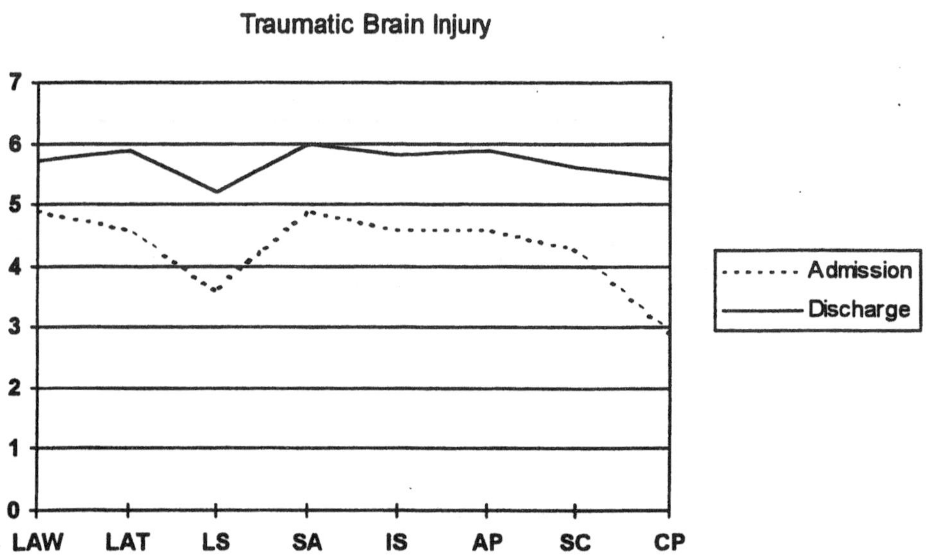

Legend:

LAW	= Leisure Awareness	IS	= Interpersonal Skills
LAT	= Leisure Attitude	AP	= Agency Participation
LS	= Leisure Skills	SC	= Social Contact
SA	= Social Appropriateness	CP	= Community Participation

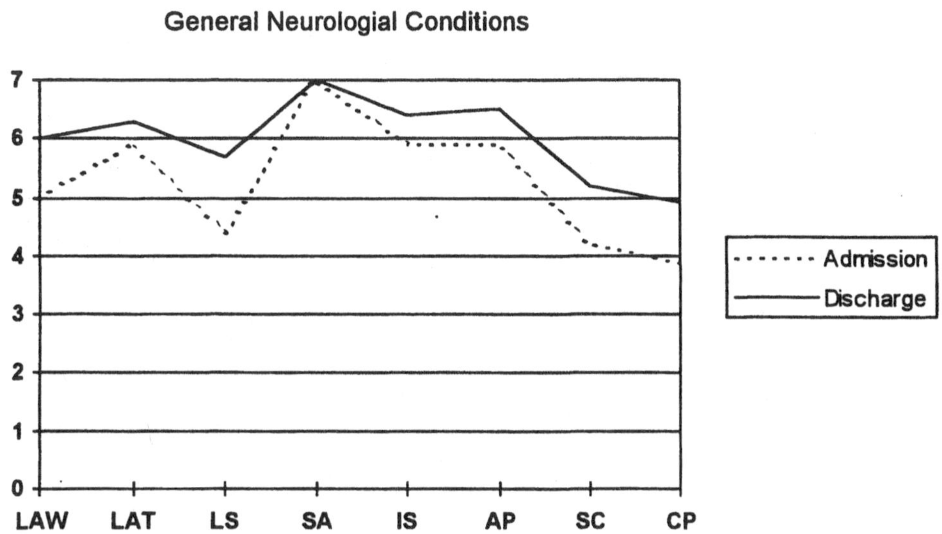
General Neurologial Conditions
7
6
5
4
3
2
1
0
LAW
LAT
LS
SA
IS
AP
SC
CP
Admission
Discharge

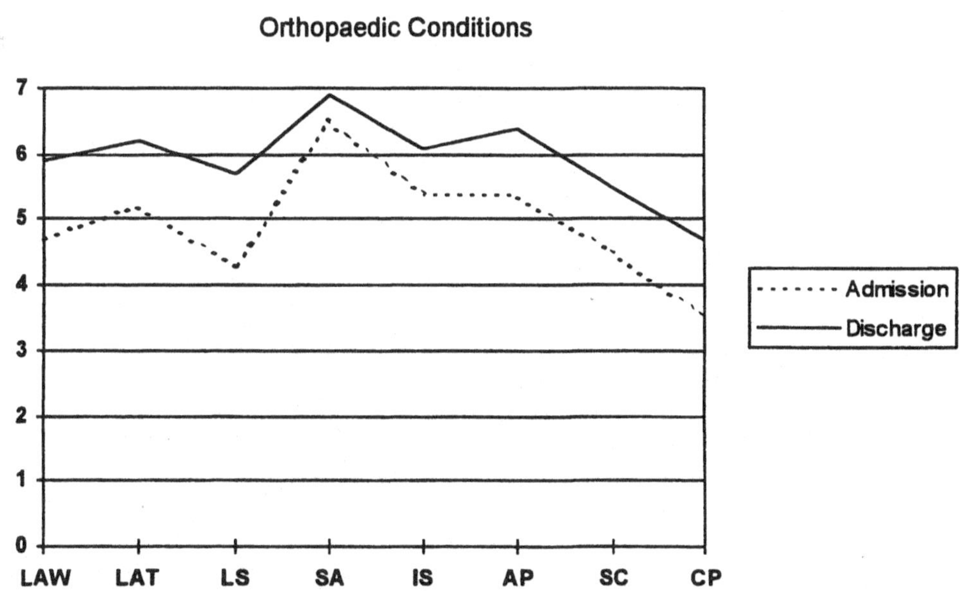
Orthopaedic Conditions
7
6
5
4
3
2
1
0
LAW
LAT
LS
SA
IS
AP
SC
CP
Admission
Discharge

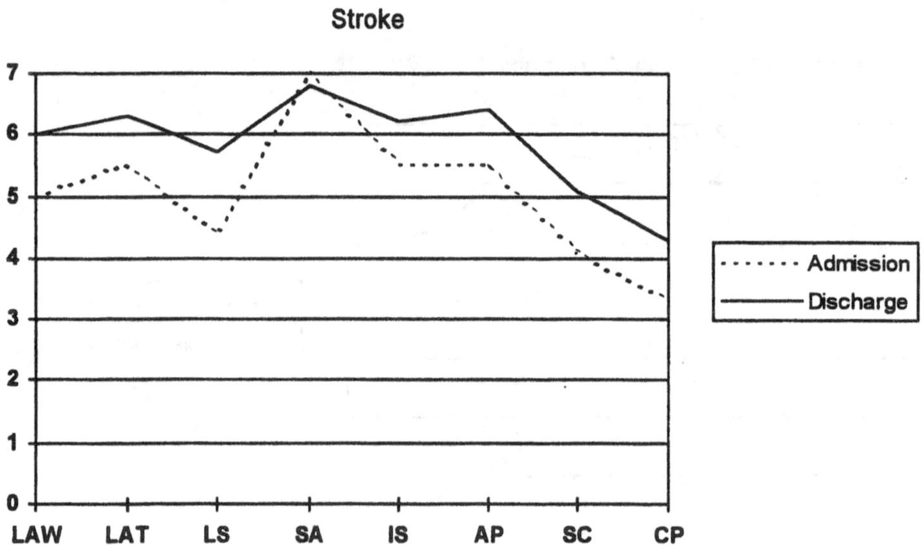

Legend:

LAW	= Leisure Awareness	IS	= Interpersonal Skills
LAT	= Leisure Attitude	AP	= Agency Participation
LS	= Leisure Skills	SC	= Social Contact
SA	= Social Appropriateness	CP	= Community Participation

Note: These profiles were based on scores obtained utilizing the original LCM subscales prior to modification. Revisions to LCM subscales included: (1) changing the title of the Social Appropriateness subscale to Cultural/Social Behaviours to better reflect cultural diversity (content remained unchanged); and (2) the Agency Participation subscale was removed and the Community Integration Skills subscale substituted in its place. All other LCM subscales remain unchanged.

Completing the LCM

The LCM is not an assessment tool, but rather a way of recording the outcome of an assessment. It is important that the assessment process collects sufficient information to allow completion of the LCM subscales, but contents of the LCM subscales are of themselves not intended to constitute a full assessment. It is impossible in a scale like this to cover every eventuality. Professional judgement is required to properly evaluate and score the client's behaviour and functioning. Experience in using the LCM has shown that the most consistent (reliable) completion of the LCM occurs when the therapeutic recreation practitioner uses a variety of information. The LCM is observer rated, and there are a variety of potential sources that should be used to collect information regarding client functioning, such as client interview, interview with family, direct observation, chart review and team discussion.

General functioning assessment information (physical and cognitive functioning) may be obtained by talking with other team members and reviewing the findings of their assessments. Personal interests of the client may be identified through an interview with the client or the client's family. If the client is unable to provide this information, or if there is limited family support, LeisureScope[8] is a tested tool that many therapeutic recreation practitioners find helpful. Standardized instruments should be used to assess leisure functioning. Therapeutic recreation tools available to practitioners and reported being used by many agencies include the Leisure Diagnostic Battery (LDB)[9], Ohio Functional Assessment Battery[10], Comprehensive Evaluation in Recreation Therapy scale (CERT)[11], Leisure Barriers Assessment (LBA)[12], Leisure Attitude Measure (LAM)[13], and the Leisure Satisfaction Measure (LSM)[14] (these are instruments reported as being helpful and routinely utilized by many agencies; this list is not meant to be all inclusive). The degree of rigour in testing these instruments varies. Therapeutic recreation practitioners should review the validity and reliability information presented by the authors of these tools and determine for themselves the appropriateness of use of these tools in their facilities, with their specific populations. To gather the most accurate information possible, it is also recommended to couple direct observation of the client with results obtained by using these tools. Once the therapeutic recreation assessment process has been completed, and as much information as possible collected related to client abilities, needs and interests, a summary score can then be assigned to the LCM subscales.

Therapeutic recreation practitioners should resist the temptation to simply ask enough questions to permit the completion of the LCM, but rather to obtain a complete picture of client functioning prior to assigning ratings on the LCM subscales. It is important when scoring the LCM that the client fulfills ***all*** the requirements of a level in its entirety. Failure to meet any of the criteria moves the client to the level below. Similarly, the client cannot move to a higher level until all of those requirements are met. If in doubt, the client should be rated at the lower level. Experience using the LCM in a variety of settings and with a variety of populations suggests that it is better to complete the therapeutic recreation assessment, then use the information gained through the assessment process to score the LCM, rather than attempting to complete the LCM while talking with, or interviewing, the client.

Not all of the LCM subscales need to be completed for all clients, nor need all clients necessarily receive a full assessment. The LCM provides therapeutic recreation practitioners with a screening component, as well as follow-up scales to assist in pinpointing specific problem areas. It is possible to screen clients to determine the need for therapeutic recreation intervention (see Figure 29). For example, the last two

(continued on pg. 85)

THE LCM SUBSCALES:

LEISURE AWARENESS

Client's knowledge and understanding of leisure.

NO HELPER

7. **COMPLETE INDEPENDENCE:** Client is able to identify personal benefits of leisure involvement. Client is able to identify own leisure strengths and weaknesses. Client has realistic expectations and is able to set goals regarding leisure involvement (based on lifestyle, family situation, financial status, etc.). Client is able to identify 5 or more activities across 2 categories.

6. **MODIFIED INDEPENDENCE:** Client is able to identify personal benefits of leisure involvement. Client is able to identify own leisure strengths and weaknesses. Client has realistic expectations and is able to set goals regarding leisure involvement. Client is able to identify 3 to 4 activities across 2 categories.

HELPER

5. **MODIFIED DEPENDENCE:** Client requires cueing to identify personal benefits of leisure involvement. Client requires cueing to identify own leisure strengths and weaknesses. Client has realistic expectations and is able to set goals regarding leisure involvement. Client is able to identify 3 to 4 activities.

4. **MODIFIED DEPENDENCE WITH MINIMAL ASSISTANCE:** Client requires assistance to identify benefits of leisure involvement. Client requires assistance to identify own leisure strengths and weaknesses. Once identified, client is able to set realistic goals. Client is able to identify 1 to 2 activities.

3. **MODIFIED DEPENDENCE WITH MODERATE ASSISTANCE:** Client requires assistance to identify benefits of leisure involvement. Client has unrealistic expectations regarding leisure involvement. Client requires assistance setting realistic goals. Client is able to identify 1 to 2 activities.

2. **MODIFIED DEPENDENCE WITH MAXIMAL ASSISTANCE:** Client requires assistance to identify benefits of leisure involvement. Client has unrealistic expectations regarding leisure involvement. Client is unable to set realistic goals. Client is able to identify 1 or 2 activities.

1. **TOTAL DEPENDENCE WITH TOTAL ASSISTANCE:** Client is unable to identify benefits of leisure involvement. Client is unable to identify any activities.

FIGURE 20. FLOW DIAGRAM OUTLINING SCORING PROCEDURES FOR THE LEISURE AWARENESS SUBSCALE

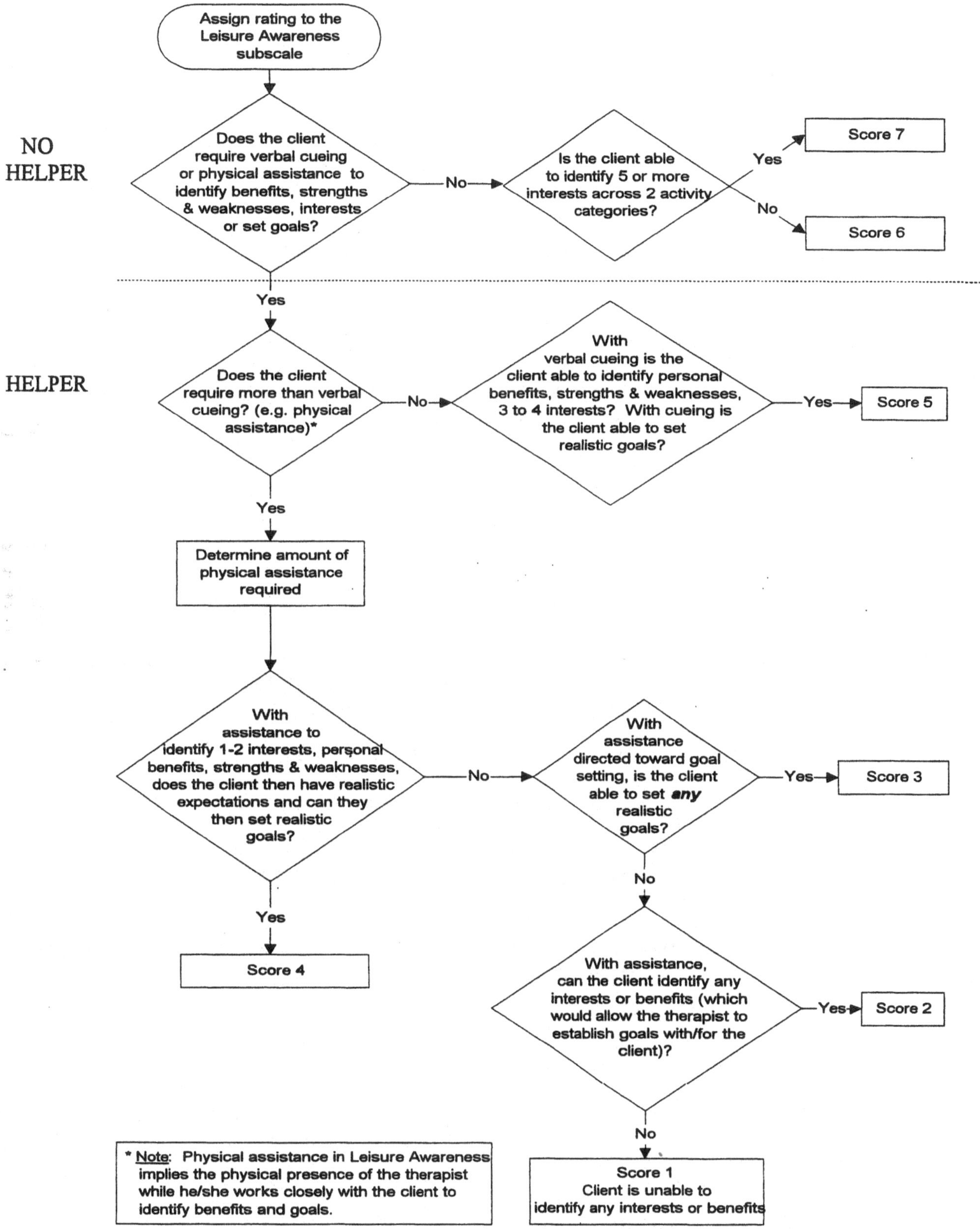

LEISURE ATTITUDE

Behaviours exhibited and/or feelings demonstrated by the client which suggest attitude toward leisure involvement.

NO HELPER

7. **COMPLETE INDEPENDENCE:** Client takes initiative for own leisure involvement. Client displays a willingness to develop new leisure interest/skills. Client demonstrates feelings of enjoyment and/or satisfaction regarding leisure involvement and participation.

6. **MODIFIED INDEPENDENCE:** Client takes initiative for own leisure involvement once a program schedule has been provided. Client displays a willingness to develop new leisure interests/skill. Client demonstrates feelings of enjoyment and/or satisfaction regarding leisure involvement and participation

HELPER

5. **MODIFIED DEPENDENCE:** Client requires cueing to initiate leisure involvement and periodic encouragement to maintain involvement. Client demonstrates discomfort with developing new leisure interests/skills. Client may or may not demonstrate feelings of enjoyment and/or satisfaction regarding leisure involvement and participation.

4. **MODIFIED DEPENDENCE WITH MINIMAL ASSISTANCE:** Client requires coaxing to initiate leisure involvement . Client requires assistance to maintain leisure involvement. Participation occurs in familiar activities only.

3. **MODIFIED DEPENDENCE WITH MODERATE ASSISTANCE:** Client requires coaxing to participate in leisure activities. Participation occurs in familiar activities only. Sporadic redirection is required to maintain client's leisure involvement.

2. **MODIFIED DEPENDENCE WITH MAXIMAL ASSISTANCE:** Client requires constant redirection to maintain leisure involvement. Client demonstrates negative feelings regarding leisure involvement and/or refuses to participate in leisure activities.

1. **TOTAL DEPENDENCE WITH TOTAL ASSISTANCE:** Due to cognitive and/or physical deficits client is unable to maintain leisure involvement.

FIGURE 21. FLOW DIAGRAM OUTLINING SCORING PROCEDURES FOR THE LEISURE ATTITUDE SUBSCALE

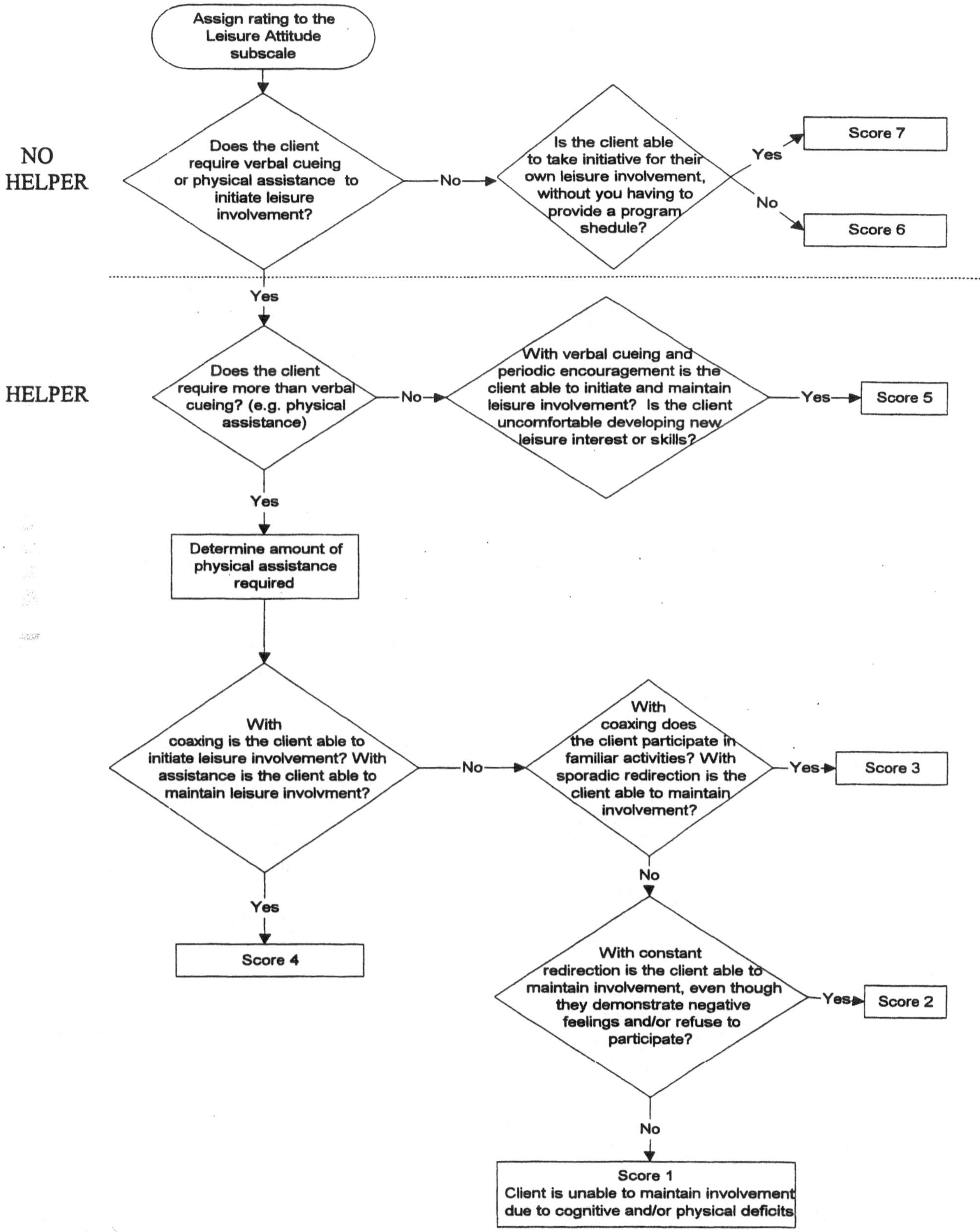

LEISURE SKILLS

Skills possessed by the client which affect leisure involvement. Ability to independently utilize assistive devices is not considered a form of dependency.

NO HELPER

7. **COMPLETE INDEPENDENCE:** Client is able to make leisure choices based on personal interests. Client possesses the skills necessary to participate in chosen leisure activities. Client possesses the ability to independently locate and utilize leisure resources.

6. **MODIFIED INDEPENDENCE:** Client is able to make leisure choices based on personal interests. Client possesses the skills necessary to participate in chosen leisure activities. With the necessary resource material (brochures, program calendars, adaptive aids, etc.) client possesses the ability to independently locate and utilize leisure resources.

HELPER

5. **MODIFIED DEPENDENCE:** Client is able to make leisure choices based on personal interests. Client possesses the skills necessary to participate in chosen leisure activities, but requires reassurance regarding his/her competence. With cueing client possesses the ability to locate and utilize leisure resources.

4. **MODIFIED DEPENDENCE WITH MINIMAL ASSISTANCE:** Client requires assistance to make leisure choices based on personal interests. Client requires reassurance to participate in leisure activities. Client requires direct assistance to locate and utilize leisure resources.

3. **MODIFIED DEPENDENCE WITH MODERATE ASSISTANCE:** Client requires assistance to make leisure choices based on personal interests. Client may require skill development to participate in chosen leisure activities. Client requires direct assistance to locate and/or utilize leisure resources.

2. **MODIFIED DEPENDENCE WITH MAXIMAL ASSISTANCE:** Client is unable to make leisure choices. Selection of activities must be made for the client. Client requires skill development to participate in leisure activities. Client is unable to locate and utilize leisure resources.

1. **TOTAL DEPENDENCE WITH TOTAL ASSISTANCE:** Due to cognitive and/or physical deficits client is unable to learn age appropriate leisure skills.

FIGURE 22. FLOW DIAGRAM OUTLINING SCORING PROCEDURES FOR THE LEISURE SKILLS SUBSCALE

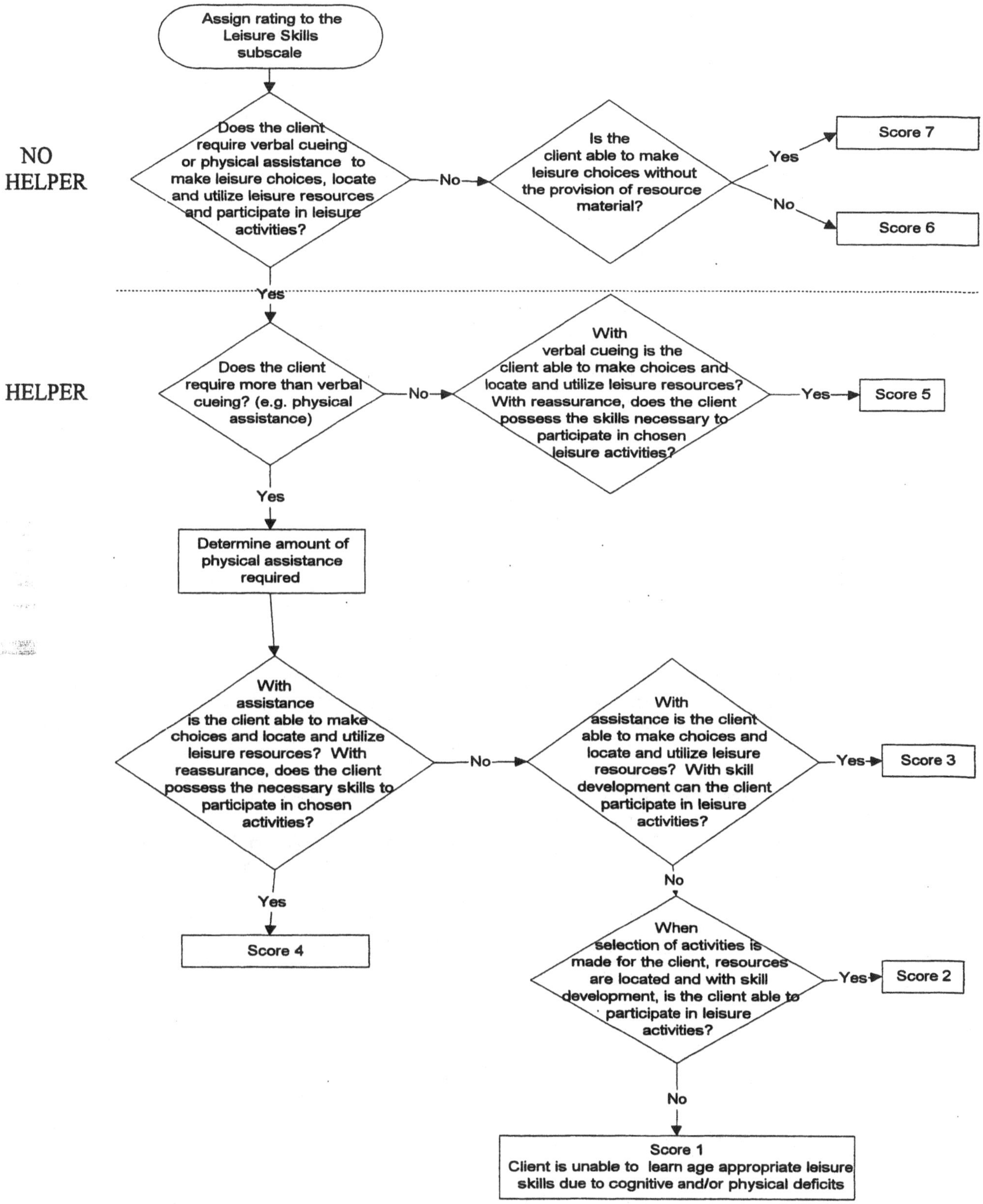

CULTURAL/SOCIAL BEHAVIOURS

Specific cultural/social behaviours exhibited by the client which affect his/her ability to function effectively in leisure activities.

NO HELPER

7. **COMPLETE INDEPENDENCE:** Client displays socially acceptable manners, personal hygiene and dress. Client is courteous and tolerant of others. Client is self-directed in these areas.

6. **MODIFIED INDEPENDENCE:** Client displays socially acceptable manners, hygiene and dress, but occasionally displays poor judgement in these areas. Client is courteous and tolerant of others.

HELPER

5. **MODIFIED DEPENDENCE:** Client requires cueing regarding manners, personal hygiene, appropriate dress and/or tolerance of others. Client questions need for improvement in these areas.

4. **MODIFIED DEPENDENCE WITH MINIMAL ASSISTANCE:** Client requires assistance regarding manners, personal hygiene and/or dress. Client is tolerant of others but may become agitated.

3. **MODIFIED DEPENDENCE WITH MODERATE ASSISTANCE:** Client requires assistance regarding manners, personal hygiene and/or dress. Client may have a low tolerance of others and becomes agitated. Client may become verbally abusive and/or display a threatening manner.

2. **MODIFIED DEPENDENCE WITH MAXIMAL ASSISTANCE:** Client requires assistance regarding manners, personal hygiene and/or dress. Client has a low tolerance of others and from time to time becomes verbally and/or physically abusive. Client requires frequent intervention. Client may be resistant to intervention.

1. **TOTAL DEPENDENCE WITH TOTAL ASSISTANCE:** Client requires assistance regarding manners, personal hygiene and/or dress. Client is intolerant of others. Client is frequently verbally and/or physically abusive. Client is resistant to intervention.

FIGURE 23. FLOW DIAGRAM OUTLINING SCORING PROCEDURES FOR THE CULTURAL/SOCIAL BEHAVIOURS SUBSCALE

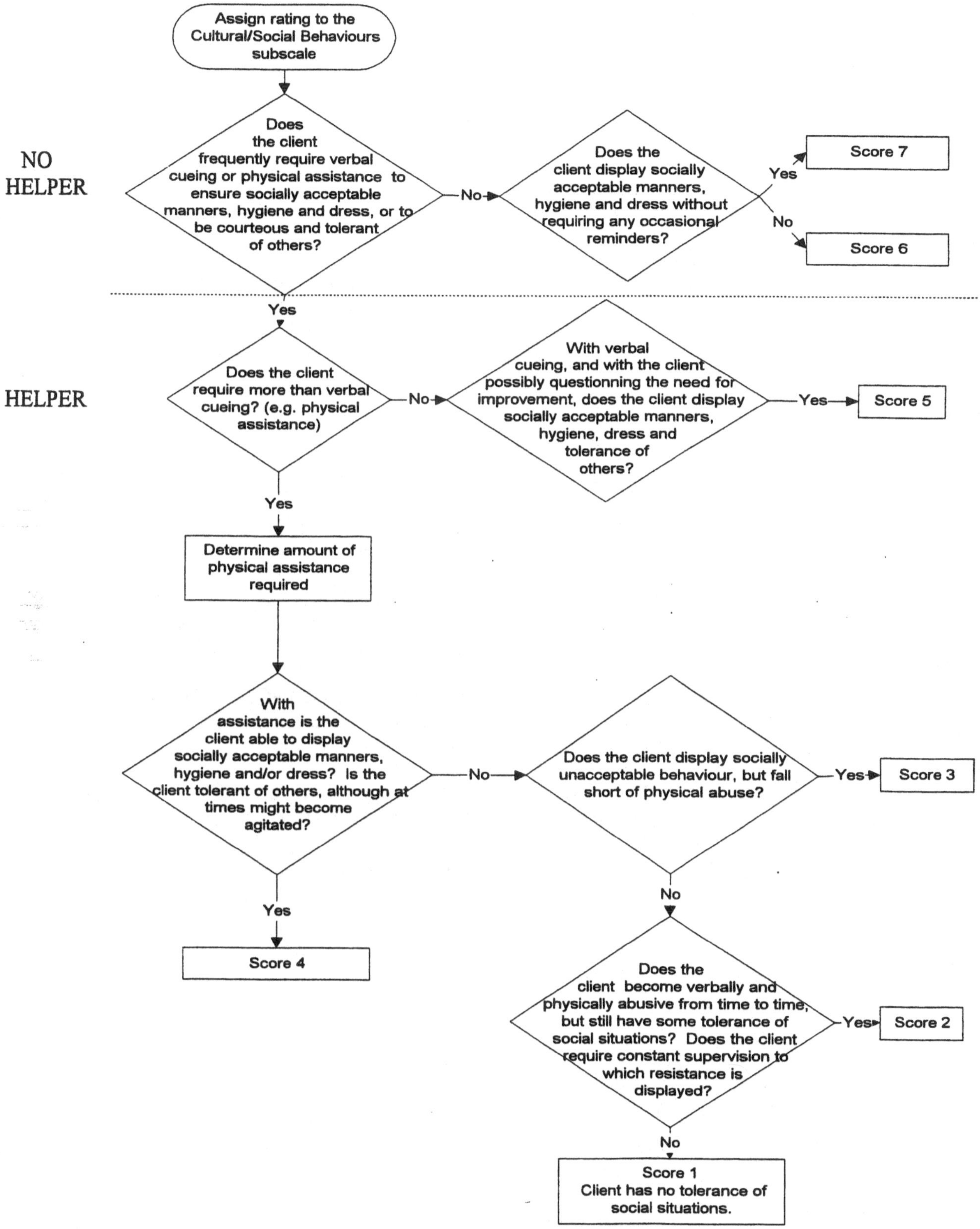

INTERPERSONAL SKILLS

Client's ability to participate within various types of individual and/or group situations.

NO HELPER

7. **COMPLETE INDEPENDENCE:** Client is able to participate independently within various types of individual and/or group situations.

6. **MODIFIED INDEPENDENCE:** Client respects the needs and rights of others within the group. Client begins to trust members of the group to meet his/her esteem needs and the client, in return begins to meet the esteem needs of others by recognizing their accomplishments, but this is happening to a limited degree.

HELPER

5. **MODIFIED DEPENDENCE:** Client is able to participate in a short term task with others, the duration of the relationship being determined by the task. Client is able to do some sharing, co-operating and/or competing. The task is the focus of the group with minimal interaction between group members outside of the task.

4. **MODIFIED DEPENDENCE WITH MINIMAL ASSISTANCE:** Client is able to participate in an individual task in the presence of others. The group is more an aggregate of individuals than a group in the strict sense of the word.

3. **MODIFIED DEPENDENCE WITH MODERATE ASSISTANCE:** Client is able to participate on a one to one basis with several different individuals. Interaction is between the client and one other individual at a time.

2. **MODIFIED DEPENDENCE WITH MAXIMAL ASSISTANCE:** Client will participate on a one to one level with the primary therapist or a family member.

1. **TOTAL DEPENDENCE WITH TOTAL ASSISTANCE:** Client withdraws, isolates him/herself from others.

Adapted from Anne Mosey, Three Frames of Reference for Mental Health, p. 202.

FIGURE 24. FLOW DIAGRAM OUTLINING SCORING PROCEDURES FOR THE INTERPERSONAL SKILLS SUBSCALE

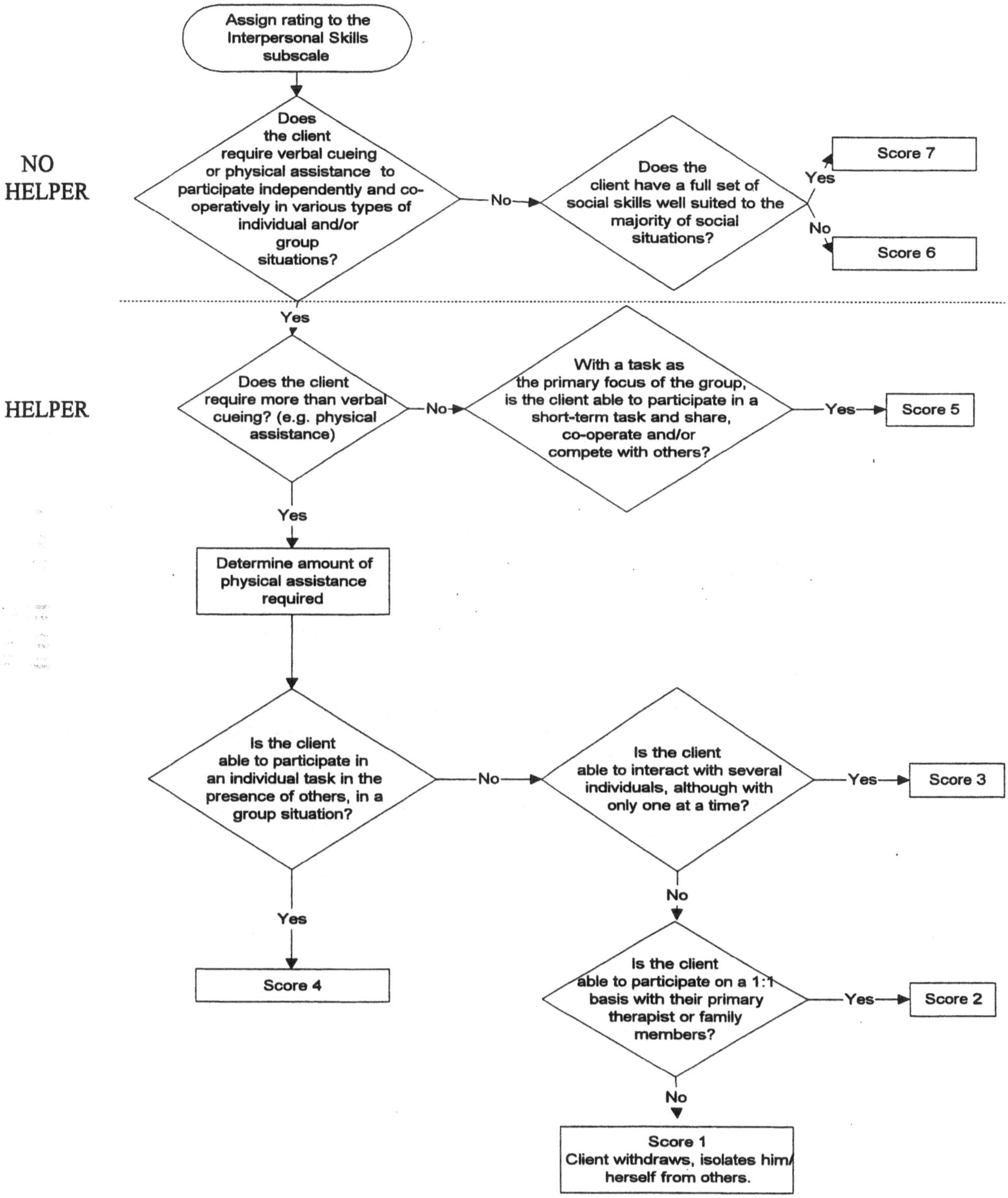

COMMUNITY INTEGRATION SKILLS

Application of antecedent skills for successful involvement in community leisure activities.

NO HELPER

7. **COMPLETE INDEPENDENCE:** Client initiates, plans and follows through with chosen community-based leisure activities.

6. **MODIFIED INDEPENDENCE:** With the provision of the necessary resources, client initiates, plans and follows through with chosen community-based leisure activities.

HELPER

5. **MODIFIED DEPENDENCE:** With cueing and/or reassurance, client initiates, plans and follows through with chosen community-based leisure activities.

4. **MODIFIED DEPENDENCE WITH MINIMAL ASSISTANCE:** Client initiates and plans chosen community-based leisure activities. Client requires assistance with follow through.

3. **MODIFIED DEPENDENCE WITH MODERATE ASSISTANCE:** Client initiates choosing community-based leisure activities. Client requires assistance planning and following through with chosen community-based leisure activities.

2. **MODIFIED DEPENDENCE WITH MAXIMAL ASSISTANCE:** Client requires assistance initiating, planning and following through with community-based leisure activities. Even with assistance, involvement in community-based leisure activities may meet with limited success.

1. **TOTAL DEPENDENCE WITH TOTAL ASSISTANCE:** Due to cognitive and/or physical deficits client is unable to initiate, plan or follow through with community-based leisure activities.

FIGURE 25. FLOW DIAGRAM OUTLINING SCORING PROCEDURES FOR THE COMMUNITY INTEGRATION SKILLS SUBSCALE

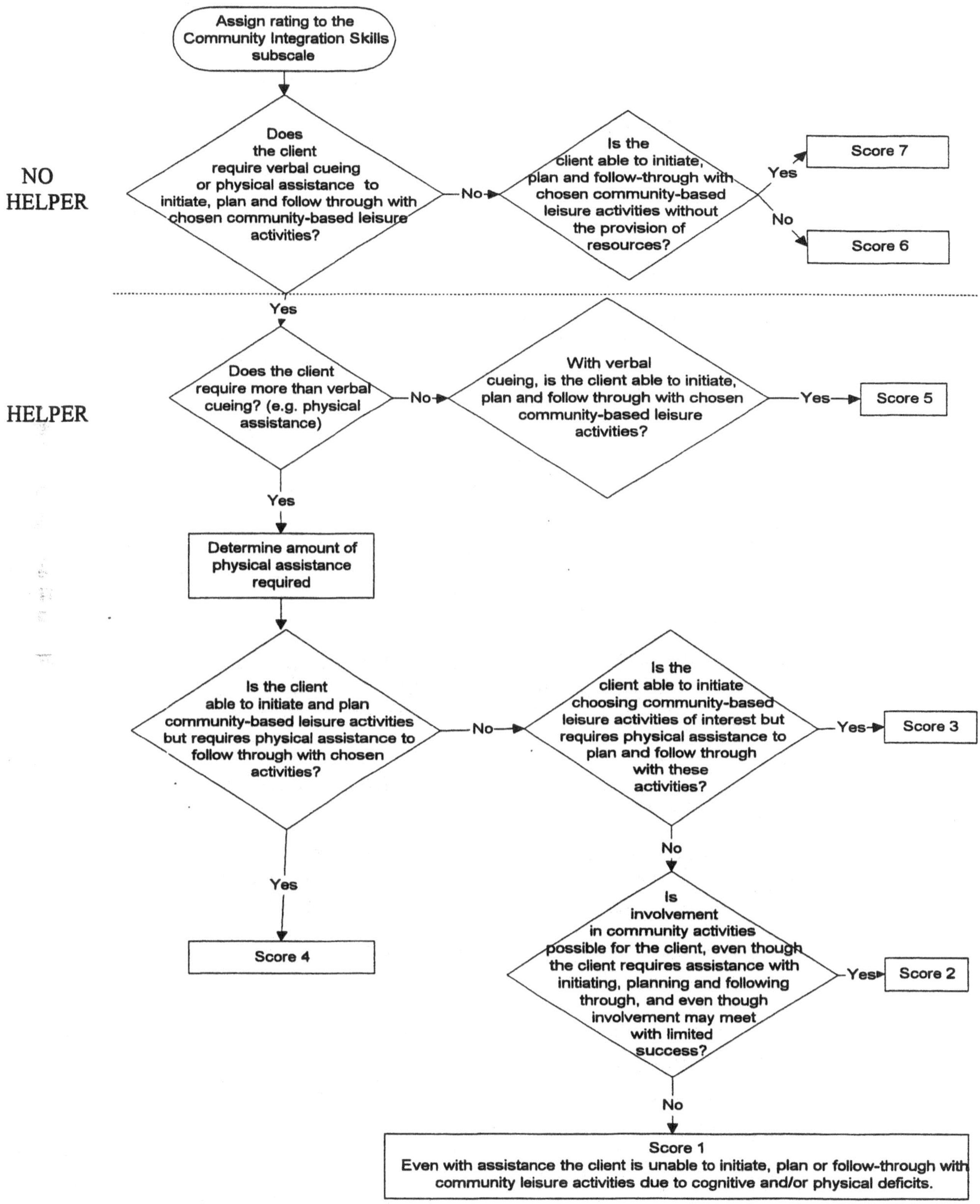

SOCIAL CONTACT

Type and duration of social contact the client has with others.

NO HELPER

7. **COMPLETE INDEPENDENCE:** Client has a mixture of in-home/community, and family/friend social contact. Client initiates social contact. Client interacts appropriately with both family/friends and others. Social contacts are of both long (>30 minutes) and short (30 minutes or less) duration.

6. **MODIFIED INDEPENDENCE:** Client has a mixture of in-home/community, and family/friend social contact. Client initiates social contact with family/friends, and interacts appropriately with same. Client does not initiate social contact with others, but interacts appropriately in response to others. Social contacts are of both long and short duration.

HELPER

5. **MODIFIED DEPENDENCE:** Client's social contacts occur primarily in the home. Client requires cueing to initiate social contact with others. Client interacts appropriately with family/friends, but avoids social contact with others. Social contacts are of both long and short duration.

4. **MODIFIED DEPENDENCE WITH MINIMAL ASSISTANCE:** Social contact occurs primarily in the home. Client requires assistance to initiate social contact with others. Social contact consists primarily of short phrases.

3. **MODIFIED DEPENDENCE WITH MODERATE ASSISTANCE:** Social contact occurs only in the home. Social contact must be initiated by family and/or friends. Social contact consists of short, 1 or 2 word answers.

2. **MODIFIED DEPENDENCE WITH MAXIMAL ASSISTANCE:** Client does not initiate social contact. Contact by family or friends is of a custodial rather that a social nature. Client may be unable to carry on a meaningful communication.

1. **TOTAL DEPENDENCE WITH TOTAL ASSISTANCE:** No meaningful social contact.

FIGURE 26. FLOW DIAGRAM OUTLINING SCORING PROCEDURES FOR THE SOCIAL CONTACT SUBSCALE

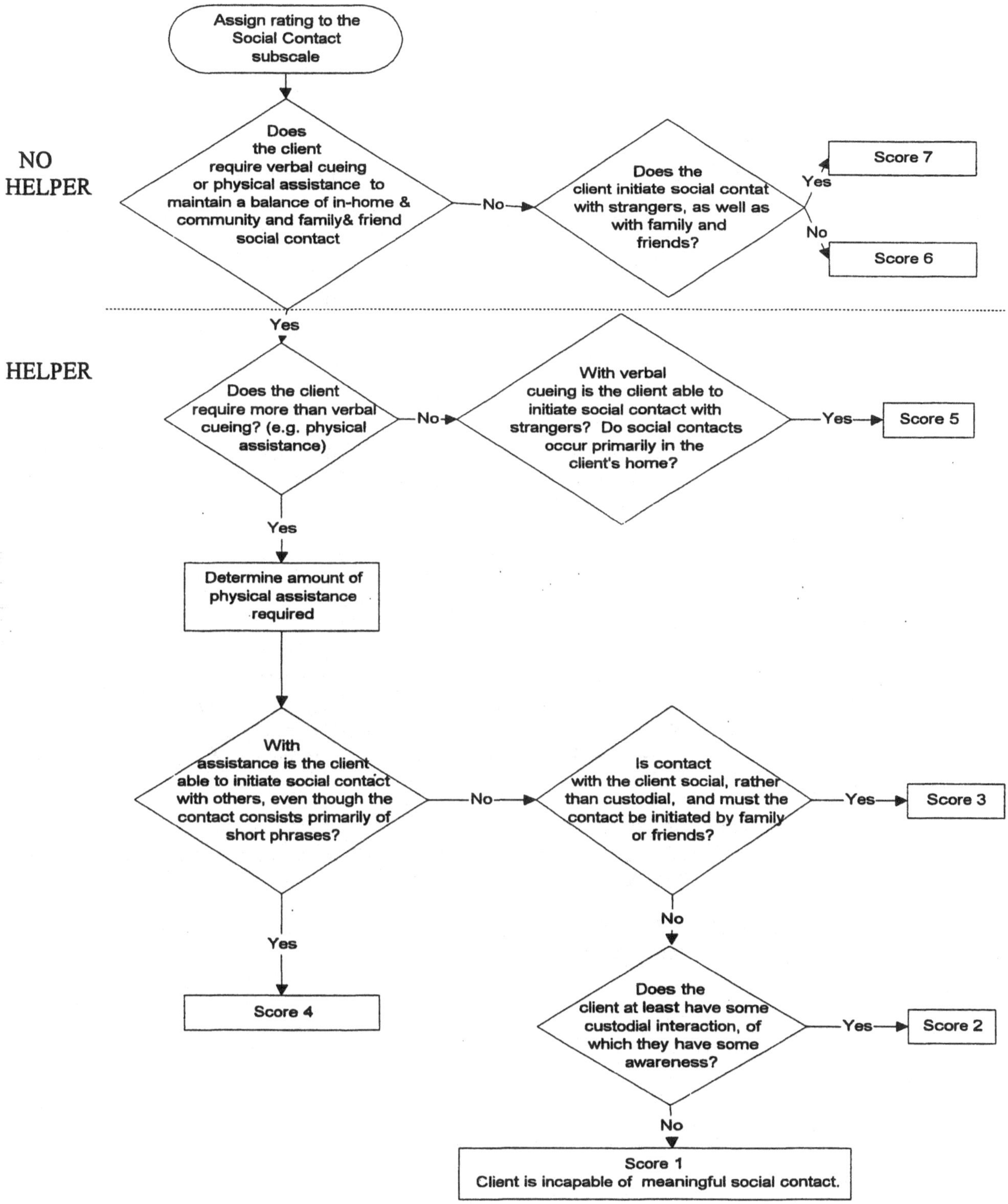

COMMUNITY PARTICIPATION

Client's overall leisure participation pattern within their community.

NO HELPER

7. **COMPLETE INDEPENDENCE:** Client leaves their home on a regular basis and participates in a variety of leisure activities. Client demonstrates a balance of in-home and community leisure pursuits. Leisure activities are both active and passive in nature.

6. **MODIFIED INDEPENDENCE:** Client leaves their home occasionally to participate in select community leisure activities. In-home and community leisure activities are both active and passive in nature.

HELPER

5. **MODIFIED DEPENDENCE:** With encouragement and support client occasionally participates in community leisure activities. In-home and community leisure activities are both active and passive in nature.

4. **MODIFIED DEPENDENCE WITH MINIMAL ASSISTANCE:** Client participates in specialized community programs. Client may require assistance with participation. Client leaves the home to do routine activities such as taking walks, shopping, going to church, and visiting family and/or friends. Leisure activities are both active and passive in nature.

3. **MODIFIED DEPENDENCE WITH MODERATE ASSISTANCE:** Client participates in specialized community day programs. Client requires assistance to participate in community programs. Client may utilize home support leisure services. Client engages in leisure activities within the home. Leisure activities are both active and passive in nature.

2. **MODIFIED DEPENDENCE WITH MAXIMAL ASSISTANCE:** Client does not leave the home on a regular basis and does not participate in community activities. Client participates in passive leisure activities within the home.

1. **TOTAL DEPENDENCE WITH TOTAL ASSISTANCE:** Client does not participate in community or in-home leisure activities.

FIGURE 27. FLOW DIAGRAM OUTLINING SCORING PROCEDURES FOR THE COMMUNITY PARTICIPATION SUBSCALE

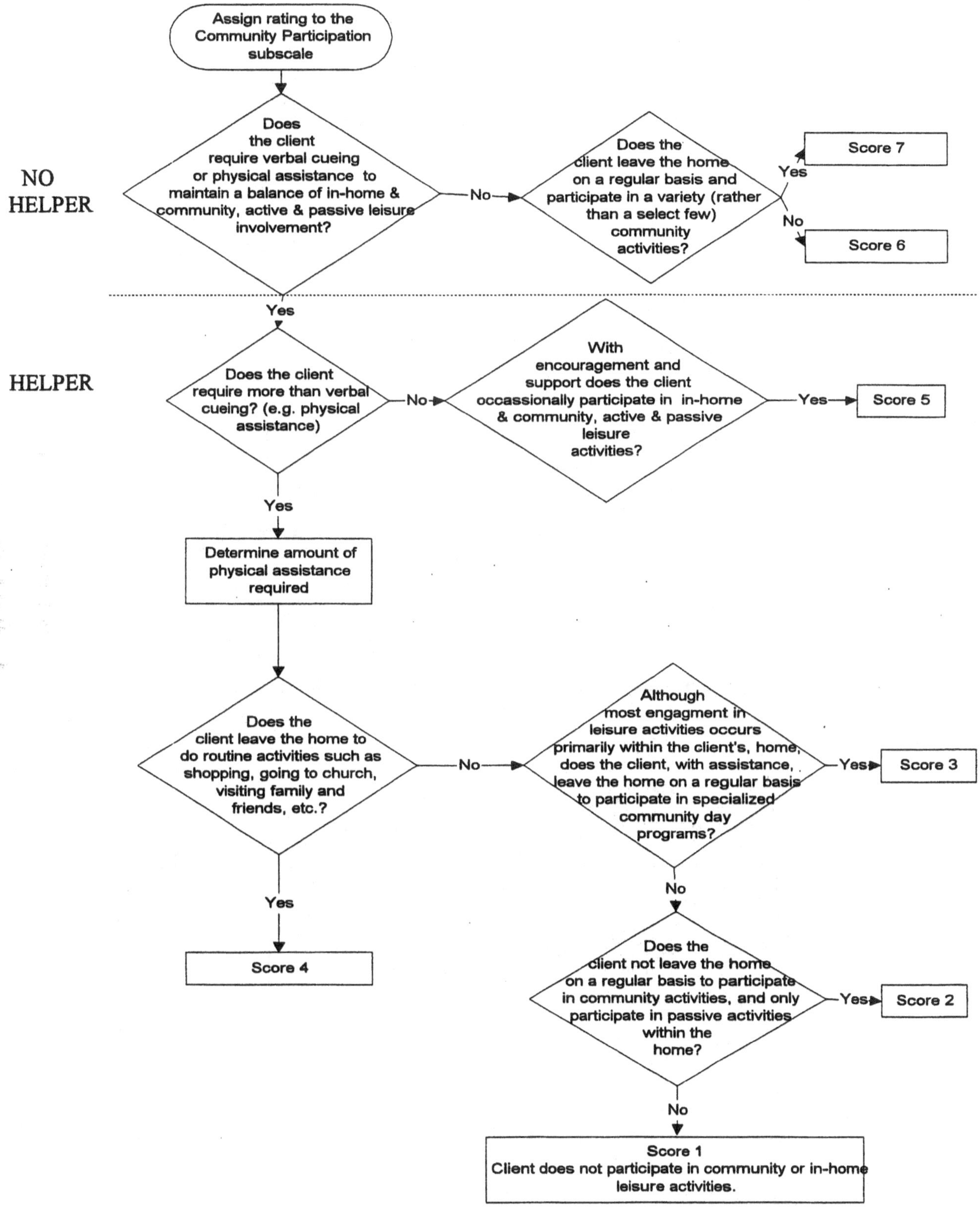

FIGURE 28. LEISURE COMPETENCE MEASURE© DATA SHEET

FUNCTIONAL INDICATORS	ADM __/__/__ dd mth yr	__/__/__ dd mth yr	__/__/__ dd mth yr	__/__/__ dd mth yr	D/C __/__/__ dd mth yr	F/U __/__/__ dd mth yr
LEISURE AWARENESS						
LEISURE ATTITUDE						
LEISURE SKILLS						
CULTURAL/SOCIAL BEHAVIOURS						
INTERPERSONAL SKILLS						
COMMUNITY INTEGRATION SKILLS						
SOCIAL CONTACT						
COMMUNITY PARTICIPATION						
TOTAL LCM SCORE (out of 56) -ADMISSION	/ 56	DISCHARGE/FOLLOW-UP			/ 56	/ 56

ADM = ADMISSION/BASELINE D/C = DISCHARGE F/U = FOLLOW-UP (≥ 2 MONTHS)

Note: Enter a value for each Functional Indicator
Enter "0" for "not assessed"

LEVELS		
	7. Complete Independence 6. Modified Independence	NO HELPER
	5. Modified Dependence 4. Modified Dependence with Minimal Assistance 3. Modified Dependence with Moderate Assistance 2. Modified Dependence with Maximal Assistance 1. Total Dependence with Total Assistance	HELPER

LCM subscales (Social Contact and Community Participation) measure actual levels of client engagement in leisure activities and the social network of clients, and can serve as a screening tool. Independent functioning on these two subscales implies balanced and independent leisure functioning overall. If the client scores at the dependent levels on these two subscales, therapeutic recreation intervention may be warranted. If the client is to be entered into an intervention or treatment program which might reasonably be expected to change leisure functioning, the LCM must be completed and scored prior to the start of the intervention or treatment program to capture a true baseline. Most therapeutic recreation departments set standards for timely completion of initial assessments.

It is important that the LCM subscales be utilized as outlined and not modified, as this will violate the psychometric properties of the LCM. The 8 core LCM subscales should remain intact and be utilized for the screening and full evaluation of client functioning related to leisure. However, if agencies wish to add subscales to address additional issues specific to their populations that is acceptable, but full testing will be needed.

Scoring the LCM (Screening vs. Full Evaluation)

The process of scoring the LCM will be illustrated by studying two hypothetical case studies (Barry and Anthony). The leisure functioning abilities of these two clients are quite different. Case Study 1 (pg. 87) presents Barry, a client with a spinal cord injury, admitted to a rehabilitation facility while awaiting placement in a facility near his home town. The therapeutic recreation specialist currently has a full caseload, and realising that Barry has been admitted while waiting for an apartment of his own to become available,decides to "screen" Barry to determine whether her intervention is required while Barry is in her facility. Following discussion with Barry, his family, the team and the therapeutic recreation specialist at the facility where Barry was admitted prior to his admission here, the therapeutic recreation specialist determines that Barry is friendly, outgoing, has family and friends who visit him regularly and whom he goes out to visit. Already in the few days since his admission, Barry has established a variety of social connections within the hospital. The therapeutic recreation specialist therefore rates him as a 7 on the Social Contact subscale. Also through discussion with Barry, his family, her interdisciplinary teammates, the therapeutic recreation specialist previously working with Barry, as well as by direct observation she discovers that Barry has a variety of leisure interests. For example, Barry occasionally leaves the hospital to participate in select community activities that are of interest to him (e.g., a community wheelchair basketball league and the local sports association for the disabled). Barry also appears to be active in a variety of in-hospital programs and has demonstrated his involvement in such activities as painting, playing the guitar and challenging some of roommates to an occasional game of billiards in the lounge. In the professional judgement of the therapeutic recreation specialist, Barry demonstrates a balance of in-hospital and community involvement, as well as a balance of active and passive activities. She therefore scores him a 6 on the Community Participation subscale, not feeling that he warranted a score of 7 because, at this point, his involvement in community activities is limited to wheelchair basketball and the local sports association for the disabled. Given that Barry has demonstrated a very high and independent level of leisure functioning, the therapeutic recreation specialist determines that Barry is not a priority for therapeutic recreation intervention.

The following week, Anthony (Case Study 2, pg. 89) is admitted to the same facility. Anthony is admitted to the brain injury unit following a severe brain injury sustained in a recent motorcycle accident. Again, the therapeutic recreation specialist currently has quite a full caseload and decides to screen Anthony to objectively determine whether her

FIGURE 29. FLOW DIAGRAM OUTLINING USE OF THE LCM FOR SCREENING VERSUS FULL EVALUATION PURPOSES

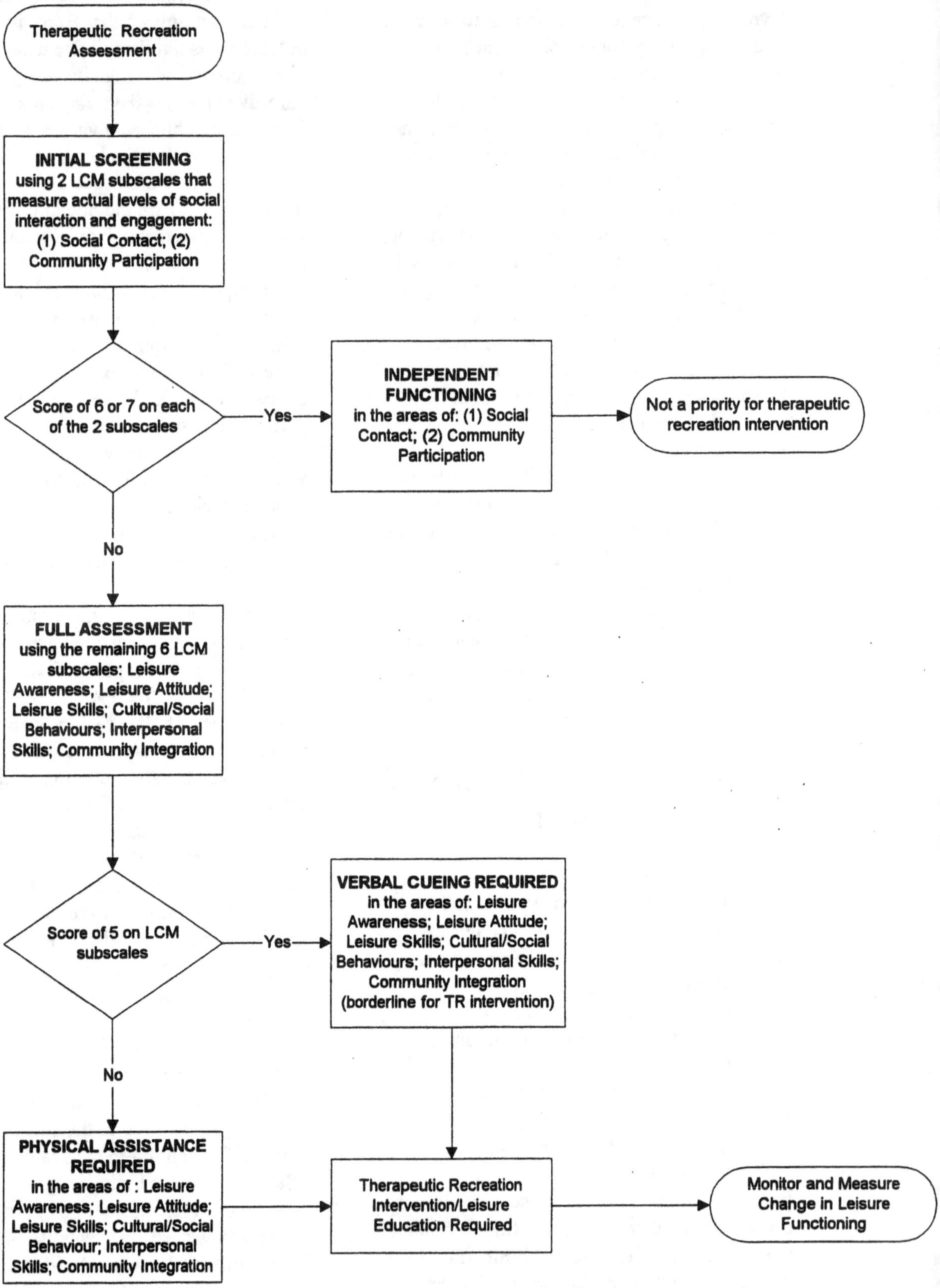

Case Study 1

Barry has been hospitalized since his car accident almost a year ago. The accident left him paraplegic. Barry has been admitted to a rehabilitation facility near his home town, to maintain his functional ability while he is awaiting placement in an apartment of his own.

Prior to the accident Barry was very active in sports, his primary form of leisure. Despite his initial reluctance, Barry became involved in wheelchair basketball and subsequently joined a community basketball league. He found that the feelings he is experiencing now are similar to those he felt when he played sports before his accident. Barry has arranged weekly transportation to take him to the local high-school for his league games. Barry has also developed interests and skills in art, playing the guitar, billiards and has become a member of the local sports association for the disabled. Barry is actively involved in many of the activities at the rehabilitation facility. He is usually the first to arrive and the last to leave. Barry has talked with his therapist about how much these leisure pursuits have been a positive influence in his life and how they have provided him with new challenges. Barry always appears to be pleasant and very much cares about his appearance. He is an outgoing young man who makes friends easily. Barry has many friends who visit, and whom he visits in return. His family is also very supportive, visits often and arranges for Barry to come home for visits on a regular basis.

FUNCTIONAL INDICATORS	ADM __/__/__ dd mth yr	__/__/__ dd mth yr	__/__/__ dd mth yr	__/__/__ dd mth yr	D/C __/__/__ dd mth yr	F/U __/__/__ dd mth yr
LEISURE AWARENESS						
LEISURE ATTITUDE						
LEISURE SKILLS						
CULTURAL/SOCIAL BEHAVIOURS						
INTERPERSONAL SKILLS						
COMMUNITY INTEGRATION SKILLS						
SOCIAL CONTACT	7					
COMMUNITY PARTICIPATION	6					
TOTAL LCM SCORE (out of 56) -ADMISSION	/ 56	DISCHARGE/FOLLOW-UP			/ 56	/ 56

ADM = ADMISSION/BASELINE D/C = DISCHARGE F/U = FOLLOW-UP (≥ 2 MONTHS)

Note: Enter a value for each Functional Indicator
Enter "0" for "not assessed"

involvement is required at this particular point in time. The therapeutic recreation specialist interviews Anthony, talks with his family, reviews the medical chart, talks with her inter-disciplinary teammates regarding the results of their assessments, and observes Anthony's level and type of involvement and interaction on the unit. The therapeutic recreation specialist determines that Anthony interacts reasonably well on a 1:1 basis with those he knows; his interaction with others is often inappropriate in that he talks excessively, confabulates and is socially disinhibited (common behaviours associated with brain injury). She scores Anthony a 4 on the Social Contact subscale. This is an example of a situation requiring the professional judgement of the therapeutic recreation professional. Anthony clearly requires more than verbal cueing to interact *appropriately* with others and requires assistance and a graduated program to build the skills required to participate successfully in small and large group situations. He therefore cannot be rated a 5. Likewise, Anthony does initiate contact with family, friends and others, and his interaction consists of more than 1-2 short answers. While he also interacts with more than short phrases (level 4), his interaction with others is inappropriate and requires graduated skill development. Therefore the therapeutic recreation specialist determined that the "best fit" for Anthony for social contact was at level 4.

In terms of community participation, it is determined that Anthony does not participate in community activities, spends most of his time in his room watching television (passive activity), and only participates in facility programs, for a short while, if his therapist takes him and stays with him. The therapeutic recreation specialist scores Anthony as a 2 on the Community Participation subscale.

Anthony scores 4 and 2 on the Social Contact and Community Participation subscales respectively, indicating a lack of independence in these areas. Barry, on the other hand, has significant and successful social contact (score = 7) and good participation in the community (score = 6). Clearly Anthony is a priority for therapeutic recreation intervention, while Barry is not. Figures 26 and 27 outline the scoring procedures for the 2 screening subscales of the LCM.

Using the LCM for Full Evaluation of Client Abilities

The therapeutic recreation specialist working with Anthony decides to conduct a full therapeutic recreation assessment to determine more specifically Anthony's abilities, needs and interests related to his leisure functioning. Following completion of a comprehensive assessment (including assessment of Anthony's general functioning (cognitive and physical), leisure functioning and personal interests (and after direct observation of Anthony's behaviour, functional ability and interaction on the unit and within the hospital), the therapeutic recreation specialist summarizes Anthony's leisure functioning on the remaining 6 LCM subscales (leisure awareness; leisure attitude; leisure skills; cultural/social behaviours; interpersonal skills; community integration) to identify specific limitations requiring her attention. Figure 30 outlines the scoring procedures for a full client evaluation utilizing the remaining 6 LCM subscales.

The assessment reveals that Anthony is unrealistic about his ability to race motorcycles again. Anthony has only identified 2 activities of interest (motorcycle racing and watching television), requires assistance to set goals, and does not know why it is important for him to become involved in any other activities. The therapeutic recreation specialist therefore scores Anthony a 3 on the Leisure Awareness subscale. Anthony requires constant re-direction to maintain his involvement in facility programs and occasionally refuses to participate. As a result he scores 2 on the Leisure Attitude subscale. Anthony requires direct assistance to choose facility programs within which to participate and requires

Case Study 2

Anthony is a 37 year old male who sustained a severe brain injury in a motorcycle race. Prior to his accident he held an international ranking and devoted much of his time to racing. He worked occasionally as a plumber to supplement his income. Shortly after his accident his girlfriend terminated their relationship.

Anthony now requires medication to control his excitability and is somewhat rigid in his thinking. He experiences pain in his lower back which causes agitation. In the past, much of Anthony's time was spend socializing and drinking after motorcycle races. The only activities of interest to him at present are motorcycle racing and watching television. He has unrealistic expectations about being able to race again and is unable to identify why it might be important for him to be involved in other activities. Anthony requires assistance to participate in facility programs and often if in a program, requires constant re-direction by his therapist to maintain his involvement. He does not self-initiate, often lacks the ability to focus, his judgement is impaired and at times he is at risk for his own safety. While Anthony does not participate for long in group settings, he does interact on an individual level with his therapist and with family members. He interacts reasonably well with those he knows; his interaction with others is often inappropriate in that he talks excessively, tends to confabulate and is socially disinhibited. In group situations Anthony is often intolerant of others and at times has become verbally and physically aggressive. Anthony requires physical intervention in regard to his manners and to dress appropriately for the weather; he often resists the assistance provided by his therapist. He requires assistance from his therapist to plan and follow through on outings to the community, and often these outings have to be cut short due to Anthony's fatigue and/or behaviour. Anthony, at this point, does not participate in community programs, spends most of his time watching television in his room, and only takes part in facility programs with direct assistance from his therapist. The results of the screening are given below and the full LCM scoring on the following page.

FUNCTIONAL INDICATORS	ADM __/__/__ dd mth yr	__/__/__ dd mth yr	__/__/__ dd mth yr	__/__/__ dd mth yr	D/C __/__/__ dd mth yr	F/U __/__/__ dd mth yr
LEISURE AWARENESS						
LEISURE ATTITUDE						
LEISURE SKILLS						
CULTURAL/SOCIAL BEHAVIOURS						
INTERPERSONAL SKILLS						
COMMUNITY INTEGRATION SKILLS						
SOCIAL CONTACT	4					
COMMUNITY PARTICIPATION	2					
TOTAL LCM SCORE (out of 56) -ADMISSION	/ 56	DISCHARGE/FOLLOW-UP			/ 56	/ 56

ADM = ADMISSION/BASELINE D/C = DISCHARGE F/U = FOLLOW-UP (≥ 2 MONTHS)

Note: Enter a value for each Functional Indicator
Enter "0" for "not assessed"

FUNCTIONAL INDICATORS	ADM __/__/__ dd mth yr	__/__/__ dd mth yr	__/__/__ dd mth yr	__/__/__ dd mth yr	D/C __/__/__ dd mth yr	F/U __/__/__ dd mth yr
LEISURE AWARENESS	3					
LEISURE ATTITUDE	2					
LEISURE SKILLS	3					
CULTURAL/SOCIAL BEHAVIOURS	1					
INTERPERSONAL SKILLS	2					
COMMUNITY INTEGRATION SKILLS	2					
SOCIAL CONTACT	4					
COMMUNITY PARTICIPATION	2					
TOTAL LCM SCORE (out of 56) -ADMISSION	19 / 56	DISCHARGE/FOLLOW-UP			/ 56	/ 56

ADM = ADMISSION/BASELINE D/C = DISCHARGE F/U = FOLLOW-UP (≥ 2 MONTHS)

Note: Enter a value for each Functional Indicator
Enter "0" for "not assessed"

direct assistance in order to participate. Without this direct assistance Anthony would not be able to take part in the activities offered and would remain inactive. The therapeutic recreation specialist scores him as a 3 on the Leisure Skills subscale. Upon observation, it is reinforced that Anthony is intolerant of others and often becomes verbally and physically aggressive towards others. He also requires assistance regarding his manners and dressing appropriately for the weather. Often he resists attempts to assist him. He only interacts with his therapist or with family members on a 1:1 basis. Consequently he scores a 1 on the Cultural/Social Behaviours subscale and a 2 on the Interpersonal Skills subscale. In attempting to determine Anthony's ability to participate in community activities, it is clear that Anthony requires assistance initiating and following through with outings to the community. Even if he does go out, these outings are often cut short because of his fatigue and/or behaviour. His score on the Community Integration Skills subscale is 2.

For Anthony, as expected, many deficits are uncovered, and begin to form the basis of an intervention plan. It is likely that Barry, being as independent as he is, is receiving limited intervention from the interdisciplinary team. Anthony, on the other hand, will have had a comprehensive team assessment. When the information is gathered the team will meet and discuss the results of the assessment. This discussion will raise many questions, such as: (1) what are Anthony's strengths? (2) what are the areas of concern? (3) what intervention will benefit Anthony most? (4) are there other general functional deficits suitable for intervention? (5) is information available on Anthony's background (supports, finances, etc.) which will allow a possible discharge location to be selected? etc.

Goals, which will include recreation and

lifestyle foci will be set, preferably with Anthony and his family's input. For the therapeutic recreation specialist, Anthony's LCM profile helps identify the areas of greatest concern and the expectations of the team will help the therapeutic recreation specialist set realistic limitations on the goals that can be met, taking into consideration factors such as the client's length of stay, the diagnostic mix of the therapeutic recreation specialist's caseload, the client's prognosis for discharge, etc. It is important to understand that sorting out many of the problems is a team responsibility. Thus, the therapeutic recreation specialist cannot be expected to solve the problems associated with Anthony's behaviour and functional limitations. Other disciplines may also be able to contribute to the achievement of goals identified by the therapeutic recreation specialist. The therapeutic recreation specialist must however, report the problem which impacts Anthoy's performance related to leisure functioning to the team for the formulation of a communal plan of action.

A number of additional case studies are included on the following pages to provide therapeutic recreation specialists with an opportunity to hone their skills in scoring the LCM subscales. These case studies, like Case Studies 1 and 2 are fictitious but illustrative of typical clients that will be familiar to therapeutic recreation specialists. Answers to the case studies are located in Appendix B, along with the rationale for scoring each of the 8 subscales. In addition, a copy of each of the 6 case studies, without the scores inserted, is included in Appendix C. These may be freely copied for intra and inter-agency practice and training in using the LCM to assist in reinforcing LCM scoring procedures and to identify any difficulties that individual therapeutic recreation specialists may be encountering. The reader should closely study the rationale for the scores obtained to ensure that the reason for the choice of score is fully understood. Accurate scoring requires a full and accurate assessment and is the main essential condition for reliable measurement. Attention to detail in both the assessment and scoring is critical. Sloppy procedures will not only produce inaccurate measurement, but will greatly compromise the therapeutic recreation specialist's ability to show significant change over a period of time. When attempting to select the level that best describes the function of the client it is sometimes helpful to look at the level above, as well as the level below the one selected to determine the most accurate level of functioning. If there is any doubt, the client should be rated at the lower level. It should also be noted that a screening is not always required prior to conducting the full evaluation. The screening option was highlighted here to assist those therapeutic recreation specialists with limited resources, who may be required to prioritize their intervention. The therapeutic recreation assessment may be done immediately allowing completion of the full LCM (8 subscales).

Interpreting Scores on the LCM

The LCM is essentially a way of summarizing, categorizing and recording the results of a full therapeutic recreation assessment. The LCM subscales and scores help the therapeutic recreation professional to simplify the complex data collected, into a meaningful summary specific to leisure functioning. In effect, therefore, completing the LCM is a step toward interpretation of the therapeutic recreation assessment.

To use the last 2 LCM subscales (7 and 8) for screening purposes requires assessment to be focused on these areas. A score of 6 or 7 implies adequate independent leisure functioning not requiring intervention. These scales were designed to be completed by any member of the interdisciplinary team. Beyond this, interpretation necessarily depends upon the skills of a professional trained in therapeutic recreation principles, the setting, the client population and the stability of the

FIGURE 30. FLOW DIAGRAM OUTLINING THE SCORING PROCEDURE FOR LCM SUBSCALES

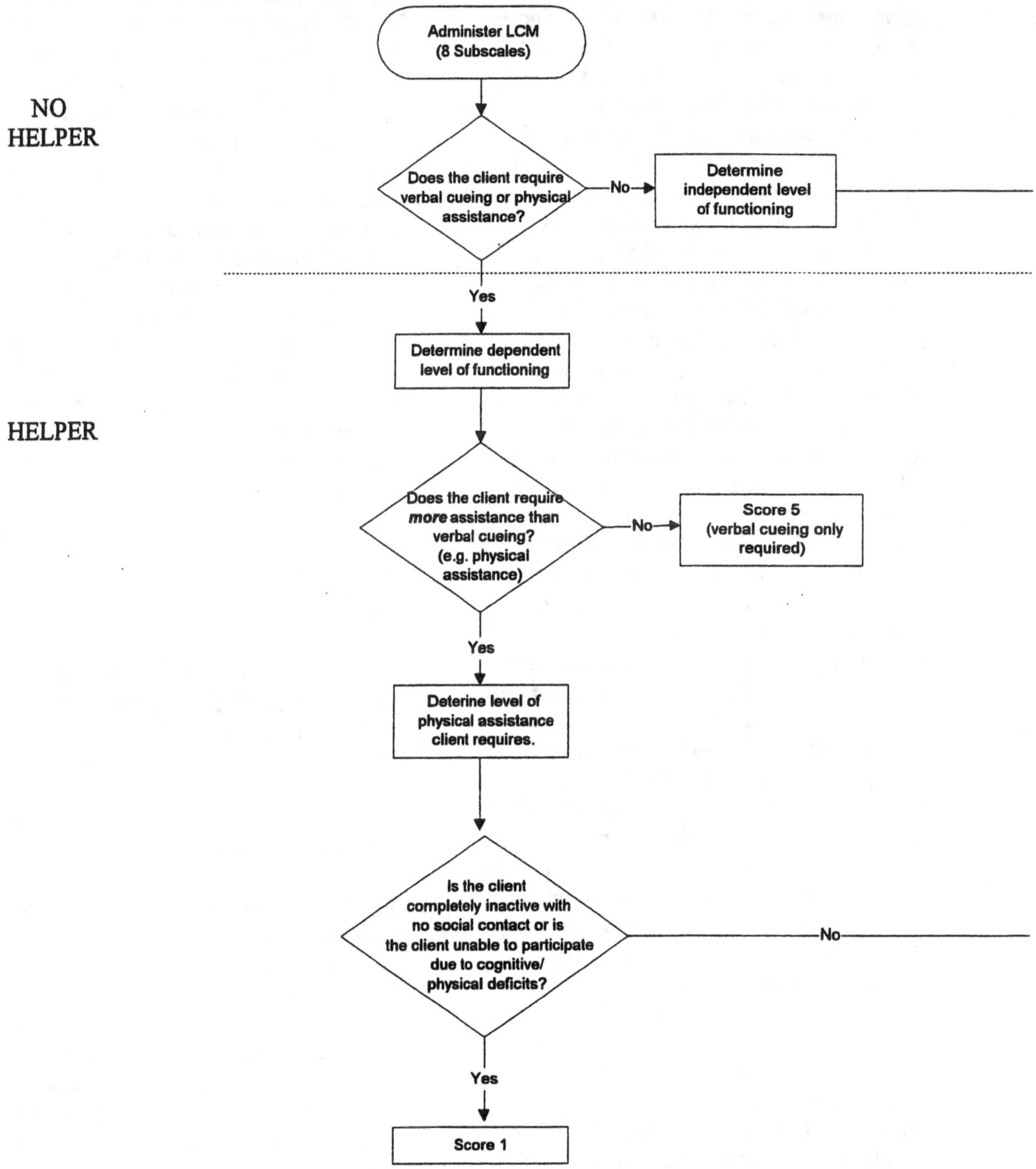

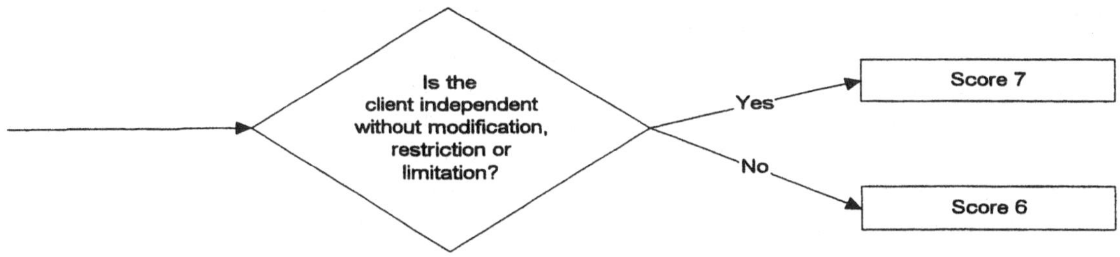

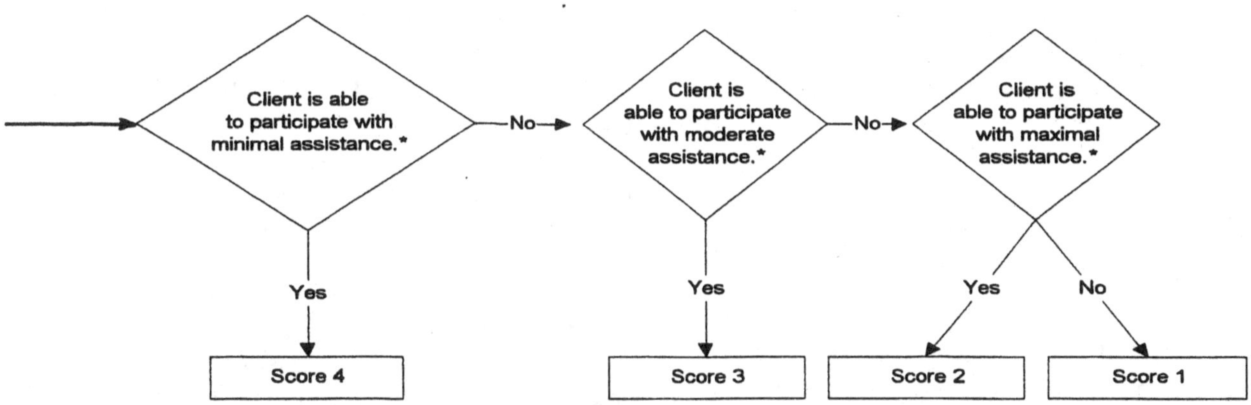

* assistance required is defined specifically for each subscale

client's condition. Thus functional limitation in a rehabilitation setting following a recent accident, injury or illness will lead to different conclusions and outcome than a similar level of dysfunction in a long-term care setting, in a stable and chronically disabled client. This leads to a consideration of norms for different populations. Norms can apply both to the current level of function and to the degree of change, either improvement or deterioration expected. How do we know if clients in a given setting and with a given condition are functioning at their full potential? How do we know if the client has shown enough improvement? Comparison with others of similar types and in similar settings is necessary and can only be done if such comparative data is available. Comparison with similar clients in the same setting will identify under performing individuals, comparison of groups of clients with those in different settings will address the issue of overall functioning of the program.

This comparative data needs to be collected and until it is available the therapeutic recreation specialist must rely on skill and experience. The necessary data can be collected through the comparative data base being established as part of the LCM system. Only when such information is available can we begin to move forward in therapeutic recreation practice and research to explore some of the tougher questions, such as linking intervention to outcome, evaluating success of a program, looking at what works and what doesn't, etc.

Is the Total LCM Score Meaningful?

The LCM, being a single factor scale,[3] of approximately equal intervals (see pg. 11), permits the various subscale scores to be summed. All of the above considerations apply to the summative score as well as the individual subscale scores. Experience and the accumulation of data on various clients and settings will eventually allow conclusions to be drawn about individual and total LCM scores. At the moment no thresholds have been developed above which function is acceptable, and below which intervention is imperative. This is simply one more area where the comparative data system will allow us to move forward.

For the moment we cannot say what a score of 38 out of a maximum of 56 means for certain clients in certain settings. However, in many team settings the total score has been used to report to the team one figure which summarizes the client's functioning related to leisure. This can be compared, for example, to the total score obtained on the FIM and for the moment serves as a simple summary score. As normative data becomes available it's meaning for different clients in different settings will become more clear.

Will the LCM Show if my Client's Level of Functioning is Changing?

As the client progresses through your intervention or program(s), re-scoring can be done at intervals which are either shorter or longer depending on the expected or observed rate of improvement and/or expected stay within the program. Re-assessment at time of discharge or other critical or meaningful times (for example, in a Nursing Home setting, when improvement has plateaued, or, if maintenance is the goal, at regular time intervals, perhaps every 3 months) can be done.

For various client types the LCM has been shown to demonstrate change (see Figures 13-18; Figure 19). What one cannot assume, of course, is that the gains result from the intervention provided, or any specific component of the intervention. Properly controlled studies are necessary to determine the impact of therapeutic recreation intervention on client functioning.

Conclusion

In this chapter we have explored the LCM, its structure, content and usage. We have reviewed the testing carried out to date and some of the work that remains to be done. It is important for the reader to be familiar with the strengths and limitations of the LCM and the settings and populations with which it can be used with confidence, and those where more caution is advised until more data is available.

The detailed breakdown of the LCM has been reviewed and its application to illustrative cases demonstrated. The reader is encouraged to complete the following Case Studies 3, 4, 5 and 6 to practice scoring and to evaluate their efforts against the analysis provided in Appendix B. We have also demonstrated in this section how different client problems can be reflected in different LCM profiles and shown how the LCM scores can change in time, following therapeutic recreation intervention in a variety of settings, with clients with varying diagnoses.

(See over for Practice Cases)

Case Study 3

Norma is a 77 year old widow living in her own home near downtown Beamsville. She lives within walking distance of the library, Senior's Centre, downtown shops and her long time friend Mabel.

Norma is in good physical health, but since her husband died one and a half years ago, she has withdrawn more and more. She used to be an active member of the Senior's Centre, going at least 3 times per week, but she has now stopped attending altogether. Even her daily walks to visit her friend Mabel have all but stopped. Norma, a once sociable, active lady, rarely leaves her home anymore. She seems content to stay at home engaging in familiar activities such as knitting, needlepoint, crossword puzzles, gardening and watching television. About once a month, Norma's daughter visits to encourage and assist Norma to put together a list of activity supplies she might need. Occasionally Norma can be persuaded by her daughter to go out to a movie. On these occasions Norma will sometimes need reminders to change her clothing and do her hair. When asked about her withdrawal from social and community activities, Norma states she finds comfort and satisfaction in staying at home and doing the things she enjoys. He says that is all she wants at this point in her life.

In the past 6 months Norma's contact with her friends has almost stopped completely. Except for visits by her daughter, there are no visitors. Norma does, however, still phone her friend Mabel once a week to talk about old times.

FUNCTIONAL INDICATORS	ADM __/__/__ dd mth yr	__/__/__ dd mth yr	__/__/__ dd mth yr	__/__/__ dd mth yr	D/C __/__/__ dd mth yr	F/U __/__/__ dd mth yr
LEISURE AWARENESS						
LEISURE ATTITUDE						
LEISURE SKILLS						
CULTURAL/SOCIAL BEHAVIOURS						
INTERPERSONAL SKILLS						
COMMUNITY INTEGRATION SKILLS						
SOCIAL CONTACT						
COMMUNITY PARTICIPATION						
TOTAL LCM SCORE (out of 56) -ADMISSION	/ 56	DISCHARGE/FOLLOW-UP			/ 56	/ 56

ADM = ADMISSION/BASELINE D/C = DISCHARGE F/U = FOLLOW-UP (≥ 2 MONTHS)

Note: Enter a value for each Functional Indicator
Enter "0" for "not assessed"

ANSWERS MAY BE FOUND IN APPENDIX B.

Case Study 4

John, an 80 year old male, has been living in a residential home for the past 4 years. He is in reasonably good health and is able to get around on his own. John attends a day program at the local psychiatric hospital 4 days per week. Although he has been involved in regular community-based activities occasionally, John has a history of decompensating without the structure and support provided by the hospital. His interests are walking, bowling, playing cards, attending plays and listening to music. When asked, John is able to identify personal benefits of leisure, but requires some prompting. He is realistic about his leisure abilities and is able to plan realistically. John is quite willing to try new activities, but knows what he likes and does not like and will verbalize same. John often states that he enjoys his leisure involvement, but requires a gentle prompt or reminder to ensure participation. John has demonstrated an ability to make arrangements for his own leisure involvement if information is provided for him. He does, however, frequently forget the specifics about an activity, such as time and place. As a result, his ability to follow through on his plans is compromised.

John is fairly sociable and likes to take advantage of community recreation opportunities. He seems comfortable in the presence of people he does not know and will converse with them if approached. John will usually only initiate conversations with people he knows. He requires reminders with regard to hygiene and dress but will follow up on his own without further intervention. John is tolerant of group settings for short periods and is able to engage in task-oriented groups. However, his conversations and interactions with others in the group are limited.

FUNCTIONAL INDICATORS	ADM __/__/__ dd mth yr	__/__/__ dd mth yr	__/__/__ dd mth yr	__/__/__ dd mth yr	D/C __/__/__ dd mth yr	F/U __/__/__ dd mth yr
LEISURE AWARENESS						
LEISURE ATTITUDE						
LEISURE SKILLS						
CULTURAL/SOCIAL BEHAVIOURS						
INTERPERSONAL SKILLS						
COMMUNITY INTEGRATION SKILLS						
SOCIAL CONTACT						
COMMUNITY PARTICIPATION						
TOTAL LCM SCORE (out of 56) -ADMISSION	/ 56	DISCHARGE/FOLLOW-UP			/ 56	/ 56

ADM = ADMISSION/BASELINE D/C = DISCHARGE F/U = FOLLOW-UP ($\geq$ 2 MONTHS)

Note: Enter a value for each Functional Indicator
Enter "0" for "not assessed"

ANSWERS MAY BE FOUND IN APPENDIX B.

Case Study 5

Paul is a 35 year old male who experienced an infection causing a severe brain injury. He has right hemiplegia and requires assistance to travel in his wheelchair more than 50 feet. Paul is aphasic but with the assistance of his therapist or family members can make his needs known. He has short-term memory deficits but is able to remember events and people that are significant to him. Paul requires ongoing help with his personal needs, as well activities of daily living such as bathing and dressing. Paul does not initiate thoughts, actions or ideas in therapy or in social situations. He has not been able to identify any activities that are personally meaningful or enjoyable for him and participates for short periods only in facility programs. Paul has a short attention span and requires constant attention from his therapist to maintain involvement. Paul becomes easily agitated in group situations but is able to interact with his therapist and his brother. Paul has no visitors, other than his brother who visits approximately 3 times weekly, for anywhere from 10-30 minutes. Paul requires assistance to plan activities. Paul is not involved in any community activities, takes part in very few facility programs, and then only if his therapist takes him; he does however take part in regularly scheduled therapy sessions.

FUNCTIONAL INDICATORS	ADM _/_/_ dd mth yr	_/_/_ dd mth yr	_/_/_ dd mth yr	_/_/_ dd mth yr	D/C _/_/_ dd mth yr	F/U _/_/_ dd mth yr
LEISURE AWARENESS						
LEISURE ATTITUDE						
LEISURE SKILLS						
CULTURAL/SOCIAL BEHAVIOURS						
INTERPERSONAL SKILLS						
COMMUNITY INTEGRATION SKILLS						
SOCIAL CONTACT						
COMMUNITY PARTICIPATION						
TOTAL LCM SCORE (out of 56) -ADMISSION	/ 56	DISCHARGE/FOLLOW-UP			/ 56	/ 56

ADM = ADMISSION/BASELINE D/C = DISCHARGE F/U = FOLLOW-UP (≥ 2 MONTHS)

Note: Enter a value for each Functional Indicator
Enter "0" for "not assessed"

ANSWERS MAY BE FOUND IN APPENDIX B.

Case Study 6

Brad is a 32 year old, self-employed farmer. He was admitted to the local psychiatric hospital with severe depression. Prior to his admission, Brad's interest in his appearance and hygiene began to deteriorate. He now requires encouragement to shower and put on clean clothing. Occasionally it has been necessary to physically take him for his shower.

When interviewed by the therapeutic recreation practitioner, Brad had difficulty identifying his leisure interests. With prompting he was able to select softball, swimming, pool and euchre as activities that interested him. Brad's general knowledge of leisure activities seemed restricted to sports and games. His family revealed that Brad worked long hours on the farm and required persuasion to take time out for himself. Occasionally he played softball, went swimming and played pool. During his stay in the hospital, Brad's involvement in recreation programs has been irregular. He tends to keep to himself and only joins in after much coaxing. Brad requires staff intervention to get started in a program and ongoing supervision and encouragement to continue participating. He usually only stays for half of the program. At times, he refuses to participate even with staff encouragement. At present his primary interest is watching television, listening to music and shooting the occasional game of pool. Brad is resistive to therapeutic recreation intervention. Although leisure education and skill development are indicated, Brad states he is not interested. Other than his family, Brad has no visitors. Family members visit approximately 3-5 times per week for approximately 1-2 hours at a time.

FUNCTIONAL INDICATORS	ADM __/__/__ dd mth yr	__/__/__ dd mth yr	__/__/__ dd mth yr	__/__/__ dd mth yr	D/C __/__/__ dd mth yr	F/U __/__/__ dd mth yr
LEISURE AWARENESS						
LEISURE ATTITUDE						
LEISURE SKILLS						
CULTURAL/SOCIAL BEHAVIOURS						
INTERPERSONAL SKILLS						
COMMUNITY INTEGRATION SKILLS						
SOCIAL CONTACT						
COMMUNITY PARTICIPATION						
TOTAL LCM SCORE (out of 56) -ADMISSION	/ 56	DISCHARGE/FOLLOW-UP			/ 56	/ 56

ADM = ADMISSION/BASELINE D/C = DISCHARGE F/U = FOLLOW-UP (≥ 2 MONTHS)

Note: Enter a value for each Functional Indicator
Enter "0" for "not assessed"

ANSWERS MAY BE FOUND IN APPENDIX B.

References

1. Hartman, D., Borrie, M., Davison, E. & Stolee, P. (1997). Use of goal attainment scaling in a dementia special care unit. American Journal of Alzheimer Disease, 12(3), 111-116.

2. Johnston, M.V., Keith, R.A. & Hinderer, S.R. (1992). Measurement standards for interdisciplinary medical rehabilitation. Archives of Physical Medicine and Rehabilitation, 73, S-3-S-23.

3. Kloseck, M., Crilly, R.G., Ellis, G.D. & Lammers, E. (1996). Leisure Competence Measure: Development and reliability of a scale to measure functional outcomes in therapeutic recreation. Therapeutic Recreation Journal, 30(1), 13-26.

4. Kloseck, M. & Crilly, R.G. (in progress). Leisure Competence Measure: Measuring Outcomes in Therapeutic Recreation.

5. Crilly, R.G. & Kloseck, M. The influence of leisure on life satisfaction in the elderly: An exploratory model. Journal of the American Geriatrics Society, 41(10), SA 50. (From Abstracts of AGS/AFAR Papers, 1993, Abstract No. P 122).

7. Crilly, R.G., Kloseck, M., Hofstede, K. & Kerr, P. Life satisfaction and leisure abilities in geriatric rehabilitation. Abstracted in Clinical and Investigative Medicine, 15, 1992.

8. Nall-Schenk, C. (1983). LeisureScope. Florida: Leisure Dynamics.

9. Ellis, G.D. & Witt, P. (1982). The Leisure Diagnostic Battery: Theoretical and empirical structure. Denton, Texas: North Texas State University.

10. Olsson, R.H. (1988). Ohio Functional Assessment Battery. Ohio: University of Toledo.

11. Parker, R.A., Ellison, C.H., Kirby, T.F. & Short, M.J. (1975). The Comprehensive Evaluation in Recreation Therapy scale: A tool for patient evaluation. Therapeutic Recreation Journal, 4th quarter, 11-20.

12. Peterson, C.A. & Dunn, J. K. (1983). Leisure Barriers Assessment.

13. Beard, J.G. & Ragheb, M.G. (1982). Measuring leisure attitude. Journal of Leisure Research, 14(2), 155-167.

14. Beard, J.G. & Ragheb, M.G. (1980). Measuring leisure satisfaction. Journal of Leisure Research, 12, 20-33.

15. Folstein, M.R., Folstein, S. & McHugh, P.R. (1975). Mini-mental state: A practical method for grading the cognitive status of patients for the clinician. Journal of Psychiatric Research, 12, 189-204.

16. Yesavage, J.A., Brink, T.L., Rose, T.L., Lum, O., Huang, V., Adey, M., & Leirer, O. (1983). Development and validation of a geriatric depression screening scale: A preliminary report. Journal of Psychiatric Research, 17(1), 37-49.

17. Neugarten, B.L., Havighurst, R.J. & Tobin, S.S. (1961). The measurement of life satisfaction. Journal of Gerontology, 16, 134-143.

CHAPTER 4

Linking the LCM to Goal Setting and Goal Achievement Analysis

SUMMARY

- *Therapeutic recreation goals should target client behaviour that can be measured, be mutually established with the client and/or the client's family, and be achievable during the client's present involvement in the therapeutic recreation service.*
- *It is important to develop measurable, behavioural goals in all settings including rehabilitation, mental health, long-term care, special care unit, as well as community settings.*
- *The LCM helps therapeutic recreation professionals set goals and monitor client progress toward goal achievement.*
- *Client improvement can be demonstrated either through gain scores or through the achievement of goals using, for example, goal attainment scaling.*
- *The LCM may be useful for continuous quality improvement (CQI) monitoring and program evaluation.*

Chapter 4
Linking the LCM to Goal Setting and Goal Achievement Analysis

Introduction

Critical processes that link therapeutic recreation assessment to outcomes, or change in client functioning over time, include ***goal setting***, ***intervention planning***, and ***monitoring client progress*** (goal achievement). Goals can range from the fulfilment or achievement of a simple task to more complex lifestyle changes. Goals should be: (1) behaviourally focused; (2) mutually established with the client and/or the client's family; (3) realistic; and (4) clearly and concisely written. The goal setting skills of the therapeutic recreation specialist will determine not only the quality of the therapeutic recreation service provided to the client, but will also directly impact the profession through others' perceptions of therapeutic recreation's value as a core health service component (e.g., through CQI reports; reports to purchasers of health services; etc.) For example, if goals are routinely set too high, failure in achieving goals is inevitable. Likewise, if all goals are achieved all of the time, they are probably being set too low, thus compromising the quality of therapeutic recreation intervention provided to the client and possibly overinflating reports to administrators and funders. Tables 10 to 14 provide examples of actual goals set by various therapeutic recreation practitioners in a variety of settings. It is assumed that each of these goals (Tables 10 to 14) was mutually established and agreed upon with the client and/or the client's family. Case Studies 3 to 6 provide therapeutic recreation professionals with the opportunity to practice setting behavioural, demonstrable and measurable therapeutic recreation goals. These cases are provided as small group exercises for students and practitioners to practice goal setting

FIGURE 31. COMPONENTS OF WELL WRITTEN GOAL STATEMENTS

Well written goal statements will:

- ❑ expect change in client behaviour or functioning
- ❑ target client behaviour/functioning that can be measured
- ❑ be achievable during the client's present involvement in the service
- ❑ take into consideration the discharge prognosis of the client
- ❑ take into consideration the case-mix of clients for whom the TRS is responsible and the amount of time (intervention) the client will require
- ❑ clearly specify time lines for reaching the goal
- ❑ express goals which are mutually established with, and agreed upon by, the client and/or their family
- ❑ be written or stated as client outcomes rather than what the TRS proposes to do with the client

and to discuss among themselves how well these goals meet the goal requirements outlined in Figure 31.

Ideally one attempts to distinguish between goals, objectives and strategies. Goals are generally viewed as larger concepts, for which the achievement of objectives (sometimes also referred to as sub-goals or sub-components) are necessary and also measurable. Strategies (sometimes called task objectives) are ways of achieving these objectives. Figure 32 provides an example.

frequency of reporting required, etc. The typical team meeting in rehabilitation settings is expensive and efficiency is critical. Inevitably a certain pragmatism is employed, as the team often has limited time to discuss the case load.

It is also important to consider the vantage point or perspective from which the goal is written. For example, as current models of care move toward more client-centred and client-driven practices, it is necessary to write goal statements from the perspective of one's client. The focus of the goal therefore shifts, to reflect the wishes of the client rather than those of the therapeutic recreation specialist, other therapists or team members, or even complying with an academic definition of what a goal should be. Figure 33 illustrates the differences in goal statements as they are written from the different vantage points.

FIGURE 32. EXAMPLES OF GOALS, OBJECTIVES AND STRATEGIES

GOAL		to improve quality of life
OBJECTIVE		to demonstrate the ability to independently attend the theatre once per month by discharge
STRATEGIES	i)	to walk 300 metres by discharge
	ii)	to increase sitting tolerance to 1½ hours by discharge
	iii)	to be independent in toiletting and dressing by discharge, etc.

In health settings, however, the term goal tends to be used less strictly and sometimes may be more like an objective. In actual practice, traditional terms such as goals, objectives (performance objectives or behavioural objectives) and strategies are often collapsed or condensed into goal statements that use more commonplace terminology and truly reflect the requirements of every day practice. For example, the term objective is now rarely used. Rather, common terms encountered in health settings include the terms "goals", "intervention strategies" and "measurable outcomes". It is simply not practical in every day practice to provide the level of "text book" detail traditionally described (see Figure 32). There are many reasons for this such as staffing ratios, time limitations, collaboration around goal setting with inter-disciplinary team members,

Definitions and terms are often used differently depending upon the viewpoint of the client, team or therapist (see Table 9). For example, the physiotherapist may declare his goal as the client being able to walk 300 metres. The client may, however, have a goal of being able to attend the theatre, for which being able to walk 300 metres (among other requirements) is a strategy. The team or family, interested in quality of life, might view attending the theatre as ***one*** measurable objective, among other objectives that are

TABLE 9. DEVELOPING GOALS, OBJECTIVES AND STRATEGIES FROM DIFFERENT VANTAGE POINTS

	VANTAGE POINT					
SAMPLE STATEMENT	CLIENT	FAMILY	TRS	PT	OT	TEAM
" to improve quality of life"		Possible Goal				Possible Goal
" to demonstrate the ability to independently attend the theatre once per month by discharge"	Possible Goal	Objective	Possible Goal			Objective
" to walk 300 metres by discharge"		Strategy		Possible Goal		Strategy
" to increase muscle strength"		Strategy		Possible Goal		Strategy
" to be independent in toiletting and dressing by discharge"		Strategy			Possible Goal	Strategy

necessary components of the broader, overarching, quality of life goal. Until these issues of definition and usage are sorted out, and they probably need to be, it is up to each team or agency to define their levels and attempt to be consistent in their usage. Comparison of outcomes in different settings can, of course, only be done if definitions are consistent.

For the purpose of this manual, and based on daily experience in actual team settings, we consider broader, large-scale goals, such as improving quality of life, as being better accepted as comprising part of the philosophy of the team, unit, program, etc. and an integral part of client-driven or client-centred approaches to care practices by all disciplines. Goals, in the practical setting are best considered as measurable performances or abilities which are important underpinnings of such things as improved quality of life, and in other circumstances are similar to objectives. The team and it's members may want to break the goal down into smaller components or sub-goals and define strategies (therapeutic interventions) to achieve these goals.

Whenever possible, goals should be stated from the client's perspective (rather than what the therapeutic recreation specialist is proposing to do), focus on those areas the client would like to work on or change, and be expressed in terms of client behaviour, functioning or performance that can be objectively measured. Goals should also include the specific level of functioning or performance required to achieve the goal. The therapeutic recreation professional and client should understand which situations (clinical setting vs. real-life setting) or under what conditions the desired functioning, behaviour or performance will take place, although it is less common to see this recorded as it is usually assumed that the activity takes place within the therapy program. If a client cannot actively participate in goal setting (due to cognitive impairment or other severe impairment or disability) it is the responsibility of the therapeutic recreation professional to ensure that client abilities, needs and interests are incorporated into the goals established for the client, to the best extent possible.

Setting Therapeutic Recreation Goals in Rehabilitation, Long-Term Care, Special Care Unit and Community Settings

The admission of a client to a rehabilitation setting implies an expectation of improvement. This expectation is framed in the goals set for the client. Clients in long-term care settings or in special care/dementia units are different, in that significant improvement is not expected, and in the latter case deterioration can be anticipated. Does the setting of goals have any relevance to such situations? Yes, it does, however the approach is different. The situation is simpler in long-term care settings where the emphasis is primarily on maximizing independence and improving quality of life. The client or resident may wish to take up new activities for which their current knowledge or skills are insufficient, providing the opportunity to define goals and, based on an assessment and completion of the LCM, determine the areas of limitation which become targets for therapeutic recreation intervention. In special care units the challenge may be similar, but over the longer term the clients or residents can be expected to decline functionally. In this situation, as well as in declining situations in long-term care, the client or resident will usually have the opportunity to participate in various activities to various degrees, depending upon their awareness, attitude, knowledge, skills, etc. as modified by the underlying disease process. The role of the therapeutic recreation specialist is to develop programs suited to the abilities, needs and interests of the resident and to make the activities as meaningful and satisfying to the resident as possible. This may require direct therapeutic intervention (as opposed, simply,

FIGURE 33. COMPARISON OF GOALS SET FROM THE CLIENT'S PERSPECTIVE VERSUS THE PRACTITIONER'S PERSPECTIVE

Goal Written from the Perspective of the TR Professional		Goal Written with a Focus on Client Behaviour
1. To increase the client's knowledge of community leisure resources by involving the client in a 6-week leisure education program.	rather	1. Upon completion of a 6-week leisure education program, the client will be able to identify 3 community recreation opportunities of personal interest.
2. To improve the client's social interaction skills by discharge.	rather	2. Within 3-4 weeks (or by discharge) the client will demonstrate the ability to participate in an individual task of personal interest for a minimum of 20 mins. in a small group situation of 6-8 clients.

to activity co-ordination) in order to achieve the residents' maximum performance. Such an approach can be defined as a goal and become the focus of the therapeutic recreation specialist's intervention and charting. As the resident deteriorates this approach may need to be re-applied to a new and simpler activity. The goals will, of necessity be relatively modest but this approach will have the effect of maximizing each resident's performance and enjoyment.

The idea may become clearer if one considers the technique of task analysis. One can describe an activity in terms of the level of skills, behaviours and participation, etc. that the activity requires. These requirements could then be equated with a score on the LCM. The activity might, for example, require all participants to score 4 or above on the Social Contact subsale. If an individual resident consistently scores much better than the activity's requirements, then the resident may be capable of more demanding and probably more fulfilling recreation opportunities. It may also be that the resident's current level of functioning in the long-term care setting, may not represent the resident's full potential. A skillful therapeutic recreation professional can ensure that residents function at their optimal level of functioning, even if their functional ability is limited.

Therapeutic recreation goal setting differs depending upon one's setting. An analogy can be drawn with house construction and maintenance. Rehabilitation is more equivalent to building a house or an addition or undertaking a major renovation. One can plan, set a budget and time lines, and the goal is clear. Long-term care is more like house maintenance. There are ongoing tasks like cleaning, intermittent tasks like redecorating and even less frequent tasks such as replacing the roof, re-wiring and even, infrequently, more major projects like renovating the kitchen. In long-term care programming, there is the day-to-day running of activities, but from time-to-time these activities and programs need to be reviewed to see if they continue to meet the client's abilities, needs and interests and infrequently, a more major remodelling needs to be done to bring programs up to date. Just as the house decorating and remodelling reflects the needs and tastes of the homeowners, so the program changes must reflect the needs and interests of the clients.

Accreditation standards (such as CCHSA, HCFA, etc.) require that programs be suited to clients' abilities, needs and interests. This implies a client assessment, an understanding of the needs and abilities of the client, as well as the design of programs that meet the needs and challenge the abilities of the client. Straightforward activity co-ordination is unlikely to achieve this.

It should also be realized that the therapeutic recreation program can, if imaginatively formatted, meet other needs of the client which may at first sight seem the reponsibility of others. For example, if the client requires regular exercise to maintain mobility, this should be incorporated into therapeutic recreation programming and can usually be easily done. Simply walking the client to the program activity room rather than using a wheelchair to get them there quickly, might meet that particular need. Clustering residents according to their abilities, needs and interests, and developing programs accordingly, is a technique that many therapeutic recreation professionals in long-term care settings employ to help manage their large caseloads.

It is usual in long-term care settings to re-assess clients on a regular basis, at 3 monthly intervals. Residents may also be clustered for reassessment according to levels of ability rather than scheduling reassessments by surname or admission date. This approach might better allow patterns to be discerned and these patterns might, in turn, help in the planning of programs. It should not be forgotten that the therapeutic recreation professional is but one of a team caring for the resident. Two way communication of concerns and successes is important and should include the resident's family as well as the physician and nurse. The therapeutic

(continued on page 121)

TABLE 10. EXAMPLE OF A GOAL STATEMENT WRITTEN BY A TRS FOR A CLIENT WITH A TRAUMATIC BRAIN INJURY

<u>History</u>:

Daniel is a 28-year old client diagnosed with a severe brain injury as a result of a motor vehicle accident. Following a comprehensive assessment it was determined, among other things, that Daniel:

- has difficulty focusing on a task and requires constant re-direction by the TRS
- has impaired judgment
- interacts and behaves with others in a way that is often inappropriate and disruptive (e.g., he talks excessively, confabulates, is socially disinhibited, etc.)
- in group situations is intolerant of others, often becoming verbally or physically aggressive

Daniel's anticipated length of stay on the rehabilitation unit is 4 weeks. It is expected that after this time he will return home to live with his parents. The TRS assigned to the Brain Injury Unit currently has an active caseload of 11 clients. The average length of stay on the unit is 3 to 4 weeks.

<u>Goal Statement</u>:

By discharge, Daniel will demonstrate the ability to participate in a task of personal interest, for a minimum of 15 minutes, in a small group situation of 6-8 other clients.

(<u>Note</u>: this represents just one of several possible goals)

<u>Comment</u>: Daniel is very impaired and his stay on the unit will be relatively short. The goal is therefore modest and, for less impaired individuals could even be considered a strategy for the achievement of greater endeavours.

? Does the goal statement expect change in client behaviour? ☑ Yes ☐ No
? Can the change in client behaviour be measured? ☑ Yes ☐ No
? Is the goal achievable during the client's present length of stay? ☑ Yes ☐ No
? Is the goal consistent with the discharge prognosis of the client? ☑ Yes ☐ No
? Is the goal feasible given the case-mix of the TRS? ☑ Yes ☐ No
? Does the goal clearly specify time lines for reaching the goal? ☑ Yes ☐ No
? Is the goal written in a way that reflects *client* outcomes? ☑ Yes ☐ No
(it is assumed that the goal was mutually agreed upon by Daniel's family and the TRS)

TABLE 11. EXAMPLE OF A GOAL STATEMENT WRITTEN BY A TRS FOR A CLIENT WITH A SPINAL CORD INJURY

History:

Jennifer is a 34-year old client diagnosed with a C-5 spinal cord injury as a result of a diving accident. Following a comprehensive assessment it was determined, among other things, that Jennifer:

- is now inactive and has been since her injury; her premorbid interests focused primarily on physical sports (prior to her injury her participation was high in a variety of sports including swimming, diving, cycling, tennis and skiing)
- has low self-esteem and self-confidence; she has demonstrated that she is reluctant to be seen in public or to take part in community recreation opportunities
- is unable to identify interests that are personally satisfying and meaningful other than the physical activities that she used to actively participate in
- is very outgoing and sociable on the unit and appears to make friends easily

Jennifer's anticipated length of stay on the rehabilitation unit is 4 weeks. It is expected that she will return home to live with her family following discharge. The TRS assigned to the Spinal Cord Injury Unit currently has an active caseload of 13 clients. The average length of stay on the unit is 3 to 4 weeks.

Goal Statement:

Upon completion of a 3-week leisure education program, Jennifer will be able to initiate, plan and follow-through with 1 community-based leisure activity of her choice.

Comment: This goal is more demanding than Daniel's (Table 10) reflecting Jennifer's greater level of functioning and independence.

? Does the goal statement expect change in client behaviour? ☑ Yes ☐ No
? Can the change in client behaviour be measured? ☑ Yes ☐ No
? Is the goal achievable during the client's present length of stay? ☑ Yes ☐ No
? Is the goal consistent with the discharge prognosis of the client? ☑ Yes ☐ No
? Is the goal feasible given the case-mix of the TRS? ☑ Yes ☐ No
? Does the goal clearly specify time lines for reaching the goal? ☑ Yes ☐ No
? Is the goal written in a way that reflects *client* outcomes? ☑ Yes ☐ No
(It is assumed that the goal was mutually agreed upon by Jennifer and/or her family and the TRS)

TABLE 12. EXAMPLE OF A PROGRESS NOTE COMBINED WITH A GOAL STATEMENT WRITTEN BY A TRS IN A LONG-TERM CARE FACILITY

History:

Jean is a 82-year old resident diagnosed with a stroke which resulted in a moderate hemiplegia affecting the left side. Following a comprehensive assessment it was determined that, among other things, Jean:

- has been diagnosed with depression
- rarely leaves her room, but denies being bored
- is sociable and enjoys talking, and visiting, with others
- was, prior to the stroke, very involved in community activities (in particular volunteering at her church, a member of the local senior citizens' centre, making handicrafts for her church bazaars, etc.)

Jean has been a resident of this particular nursing home for 3 years. Her husband visits 3-4 times weekly, and usually stays anywhere from 1 to 2 hours each visit. Jean's husband is concerned that Jean is becoming withdrawn and he is worried about her depression.

Combined Progress Note & Goal Statement:

Level of Involvement Jean continues to remain in her room, content to follow her own daily routine of watching her favourite television programs, writing letters to her children, grandchildren and family, and knitting. She only leaves her room for meals, 1x/week to attend church, 1x/every 2 weeks to get her hair done and occasionally to go for a walk in the garden with her husband. 10-15 minutes are spent daily inviting her to join activities with other residents.

Behaviour Jean refuses to leave her room, stating she is happy with her daily routine. However, she always welcomes staff to sit and visit with her in her room.

Goal/Plan Will spend 15-20 mins./week with resident in her room reviewing her activities, discussing recent events and encouraging fuller participation in the activities of the home.

		Yes	No
?	Does the goal statement expect change in client behaviour?	☐	☑
?	Can the change in client behaviour be measured?	☐	☑
?	Is the goal achievable during the client's present length of stay?	☑	☐
?	Is the goal consistent with the discharge prognosis of the client?	☑	☐
?	Is the goal feasible given the case-mix of the TRS?	☑	☐
?	Does the goal clearly specify time lines for reaching the goal?	☐	☑
?	Is the goal written in a way that reflects *client* outcomes? (it is assumed that the goal was mutually agreed upon by Jean, her husband and the TRS)	☐	☑

Comment: The goals developed for Jean do not meet all the criteria for goal setting. There is no clear expectation of change in behaviour and the goals are written from the perspective of what the TRS, not Jean, will do. As there are no specific outcomes, there are no specific time lines. The goal for Jean that could improve matters is that Jean will, during the next four months, begin and continue to attend one program held outside of her room. The TRS could also plan to discuss her observations regarding the concerns the client is raising with nursing staff and the physician to ensure that the possibility of depression is considered.

TABLE 13. EXAMPLE OF A PROGRESS NOTE COMBINED WITH A GOAL STATEMENT WRITTEN BY A TRS IN A LONG-TERM CARE FACILITY

History:

Harold is a 79-year old resident diagnosed with Parkinson's Disease and mild cognitive impairment. Following a comprehensive assessment it was determined, among other things, that Harold:

- has difficulty with fine motor co-ordination
- has problems with short-term memory but compensates well
- is sociable and outgoing but has limited tolerance, tiring easily
- previously was physically active enjoying golf and sailing

Harold has been a resident of this residential home for approximately 6 years.

Combined Progress Note & Goal Statement:

Level of Involvement **Behaviour**	Harold continues to participate in 3 to 4 activities every day (see attendance chart). Occasionally (1-2x/month) becomes agitated when he requires assistance (e.g., calling family; problems with friend Martha). Harold regularly attends programs offered although frequently needs reminding. In group situations he is socially appropriate and participates well although the Parkinson's Disease has reduced his voice volume which is a limitation. He plays cards with the use of a card holder, needed because of tremor, but has some difficulty keeping track of the cards. He would like to be physically more active but isn't sure he can achieve much more.
Goal	Harold will maintain his level of socialization by continuing with the card group, and improve his memory through mental stimulation and memory work. Over the next 3 months Harold will improve his fitness and tolerance by gradually increasing his participation in more physically active programs.
Plan	Will explore the possibility of his participating in the bowling group. Will discuss medications with physician as Harold seems to fluctuate significantly. If this is related to when the medication is given, would it be helpful to take the medication shortly before bowling time? As the physiotherapist feels activity will help maintain Harold's mobility TRS will walk him to the activity programs each day.

? Does the goal statement expect change in client behaviour? ☑ Yes ☐ No
? Can the change in client behaviour be measured? ☑ Yes ☐ No
? Is the goal achievable during the client's present length of stay? ☑ Yes ☐ No
? Is the goal consistent with the discharge prognosis of the client? ☑ Yes ☐ No
? Is the goal feasible given the case-mix of the TRS? ☑ Yes ☐ No
? Does the goal clearly specify time lines for reaching the goal? ☑ Yes ☐ No
? Is the goal written in a way that reflects ***client*** outcomes? ☑ Yes ☐ No
(it is assumed that the goal was mutually agreed upon by Harold and/or his family and the TRS)

TABLE 14. EXAMPLE OF A PROGRESS NOTE COMBINED WITH A GOAL STATEMENT WRITTEN BY A TRS IN A SPECIAL CARE/DEMENTIA UNIT.

History:

Helen is a 73-year old resident of a special care dementia unit. She has a diagnosis of Alzheimer Disease. Following a comprehensive assessment it was determined that, among other things, Helen:

- has moderate cognitive impairment (MMSE=15)
- tends to wander and get lost
- can be disruptive at night but settles better if she has been physically active through the day
- has limited attention span, losing interest after a few minutes and requiring much re-direction and encouragement

Helen has been a resident of this residential home for approximately 6 months. It is unclear what Helen's previous interests were. She is unable to provide the TRS with this information and her family is unsupportive.

Combined Progress Note & Goal Statement:

Level of Involvement	Helen attends recreation programs daily. A volunteer from her church takes her out once a week for a car ride, and also occasionally for a meal.
Behaviour	Helen's limited attention span makes it difficult for her to attend to a program for more that 5 to 10 mins., although with constant re-direction and encouragement she can remain involved for up to 15 to 20 mins. She walks a great deal around the unit and enjoys going with the group into the gardens but requires close supervision. She seems more content when physically active, but also responds well to the presence of others in a group situation. In the current events group however she seems distracted and unable to participate actively.
Goal	Helen will continue involvement in group settings to attempt to maintain social skills. She will attend the reminiscent group as she seems to enjoy listening to the stories of others and might be encouraged to participate. Her LCM scores suggest that although she scores very poorly on most LCM subscales she has sufficient interpersonal skills to participate in this group. She will cease to attend the current events group. Helen will have increased physical activity through involvement in the walking and exercise groups. The effect of this on night-time agitation and sleeping will be monitored.

Question	Yes	No
? Does the goal statement expect change in client behaviour?	☑ Yes	☐ No
? Can the change in client behaviour be measured?	☑ Yes	☐ No
? Is the goal achievable during the client's present length of stay?	☑ Yes	☐ No
? Is the goal consistent with the discharge prognosis of the client?	☑ Yes	☐ No
? Is the goal feasible given the case-mix of the TRS?	☑ Yes	☐ No
? Does the goal clearly specify time lines for reaching the goal?	☐ Yes	☑ No
? Is the goal written in a way that reflects *client* outcomes?	☑ Yes	☐ No

Practice Case Studies:

Case Study 3

Norma is a 77 year old widow living in her own home near downtown Beamsville. She lives within walking distance of the library, Senior's Centre, downtown shops and her long time friend Mabel.

Norma is in good physical health, but since her husband died one and a half years ago, she has withdrawn more and more. She used to be an active member of the Senior's Centre, going at least 3 times per week, but she has now stopped attending altogether. Even her daily walks to visit her friend Mabel have all but stopped. Norma, a once sociable, active lady, rarely leaves her home anymore. She seems content to stay at home engaging in familiar activities such as knitting, needlepoint, crossword puzzles, gardening and watching television. About once a month, Norma's daughter visits to encourage and assist Norma to put together a list of activity supplies she might need. Occasionally Norma can be persuaded by her daughter to go out to a movie. On these occasions Norma will sometimes need reminders to change her clothing and do her hair. When asked about her withdrawal from social and community activities, Norma states she finds comfort and satisfaction in staying at home and doing the things she enjoys. She says that is all she wants at this point in her life.

In the past 6 months Norma's contact with her friends has almost stopped completely. Except for visits by her daughter, there are no visitors. Norma does, however, still phone her friend Mabel once a week to talk about old times.

Hypothetical Goal Statement:

____

____

____

____

____

____

Does the goal statement expect change in client behaviour?	❑ Yes	❑ No
Can the change in client behaviour be measured?	❑ Yes	❑ No
Is the goal achievable during the client's present length of stay?	❑ Yes	❑ No
Is the goal consistent with the discharge prognosis of the client?	❑ Yes	❑ No
Is the goal feasible given the case-mix of the TRS?	❑ Yes	❑ No
Does the goal clearly specify time lines for reaching the goal?	❑ Yes	❑ No
Is the goal written in a way that reflects ***client*** outcomes?	❑ Yes	❑ No
Was the goal discussed with the client and/or client's family?	❑ Yes	❑ No

Case Study 4

John, an 80 year old male, has been living in a residential home for the past 4 years. He is in reasonably good health and is able to get around on his own. John attends a day program at the local psychiatric hospital 4 days per week. Although he has been involved in regular community-based activities occasionally, John has a history of decompensating without the structure and support provided by the hospital. His interests are walking, bowling, playing cards, attending plays and listening to music. When asked, John is able to identify personal benefits of leisure, but requires some prompting. He is realistic about his leisure abilities and is able to plan realistically. John is quite willing to try new activities, but knows what he likes and does not like and will verbalize same. John often states that he enjoys his leisure involvement, but requires a gentle prompt or reminder to ensure participation. John has demonstrated an ability to make arrangements for his own leisure involvement if information is provided for him. He does, however, frequently forget the specifics about an activity, such as time and place. As a result, his ability to follow through on his plans is compromised.

John is fairly sociable and likes to take advantage of community recreation opportunities. He seems comfortable in the presence of people he does not know and will converse with them if approached. John will usually only initiate conversations with people he knows. He requires reminders with regard to hygiene and dress but will follow up on his own without further intervention. John is tolerant of group settings for short periods and is able to engage in task-oriented groups. However, his conversations and interactions with others in the group are limited.

Hypothetical Goal Statement:

____

____

____

____

____

____

____

Does the goal statement expect change in client behaviour?	❑ Yes	❑ No
Can the change in client behaviour be measured?	❑ Yes	❑ No
Is the goal achievable during the client's present length of stay?	❑ Yes	❑ No
Is the goal consistent with the discharge prognosis of the client?	❑ Yes	❑ No
Is the goal feasible given the case-mix of the TRS?	❑ Yes	❑ No
Does the goal clearly specify time lines for reaching the goal?	❑ Yes	❑ No
Is the goal written in a way that reflects *client* outcomes?	❑ Yes	❑ No
Was the goal discussed with the client and/or client's family?	❑ Yes	❑ No

Case Study 5

Paul is a 35 year old male who experienced an infection causing a severe brain injury. He has a right hemiplegia and requires assistance to travel in his wheelchair more than 50 feet. Paul is aphasic but with the assistance of his therapist or family members can make his needs known. He has short-term memory deficits but is able to remember events and people that are significant to him. Paul requires ongoing help with his personal needs, as well as with activities of daily living such as bathing and dressing. Paul does not initiate thoughts, actions or ideas in therapy or in social situations. He has not been able to identify any activities that are personally meaningful or enjoyable for him and participates for short periods only in facility programs. Paul has a short attention span and requires constant attention from his therapist to maintain involvement. Paul becomes easily agitated in group situations but is able to interact with his therapist and his brother. Paul has no visitors, other than his brother who visits approximately 3 times weekly, for anywhere from 10-30 minutes. Paul requires assistance to plan activities. Paul is not involved in any community activities, takes part in very few facility programs, and then only if his therapist takes him; he does however take part in regularly scheduled therapy sessions.

Hypothetical Goal Statement:

____

____

____

____

____

____

____

Does the goal statement expect change in client behaviour?	❑ Yes	❑ No
Can the change in client behaviour be measured?	❑ Yes	❑ No
Is the goal achievable during the client's present length of stay?	❑ Yes	❑ No
Is the goal consistent with the discharge prognosis of the client?	❑ Yes	❑ No
Is the goal feasible given the case-mix of the TRS?	❑ Yes	❑ No
Does the goal clearly specify time lines for reaching the goal?	❑ Yes	❑ No
Is the goal written in a way that reflects ***client*** outcomes?	❑ Yes	❑ No
Was the goal discussed with the client and/or client's family?	❑ Yes	❑ No

Case Study 6

Brad is a 32 year old, self-employed farmer. He was admitted to the local psychiatric hospital with severe depression. Prior to his admission, Brad's interest in his appearance and hygiene began to deteriorate. He now requires encouragement to shower and put on clean clothing. Occasionally it has been necessary to physically take him for his shower.

When interviewed by the therapeutic recreation practitioner, Brad had difficulty identifying his leisure interests. With prompting he was able to select softball, swimming, pool and euchre as activities that interested him. Brad's general knowledge of leisure activities seemed restricted to sports and games. His family revealed that Brad worked long hours on the farm and required persuasion to take time out for himself. Occasionally he played softball, went swimming and played pool. During his stay in the hospital, Brad's involvement in recreation programs has been irregular. He tends to keep to himself and only joins in after much coaxing. Brad requires staff intervention to get started in a program and ongoing supervision and encouragement to continue participating. He usually only stays for half of the program. At times, he refuses to participate even with staff encouragement. At present his primary interest is watching television, listening to music and shooting the occasional game of pool. Brad is resistive to therapeutic recreation intervention. Although leisure education and skill development are indicated, Brad states he is not interested. Other than his family, Brad has no visitors. Family members visit approximately 3-5 times per week for approximately 1-2 hours at a time.

Hypothetical Goal Statement:

Does the goal statement expect change in client behaviour?	❑ Yes	❑ No
Can the change in client behaviour be measured?	❑ Yes	❑ No
Is the goal achievable during the client's present length of stay?	❑ Yes	❑ No
Is the goal consistent with the discharge prognosis of the client?	❑ Yes	❑ No
Is the goal feasible given the case-mix of the TRS?	❑ Yes	❑ No
Does the goal clearly specify time lines for reaching the goal?	❑ Yes	❑ No
Is the goal written in a way that reflects ***client*** outcomes?	❑ Yes	❑ No
Was the goal discussed with the client and/or client's family?	❑ Yes	❑ No

recreation specialist might notice the client is over sedated, tired or depressed or that some unexpected deterioration has occurred. This observation should be shared. The family can also provide valuable input about the client's tastes and preferences and the client might be more willing to share concerns with the family than the therapeutic recreation specialist. The therapeutic recreation specialist should remember that the family's desire to be involved is not only understandable but desirable and to be encouraged. For clients continuing to live in the community similar approaches can be applied depending upon whether the client is seen more for rehabilitation or maintenance. The same principles of goal setting apply whatever the setting, and the same need to demonstrate outcomes to justify service applies. The goal in long-term care for a stable client is to design activities which reflect the abilities of the client, rather than, as in rehabilitation, improve the client to meet the challenges of the activity.

Setting Goals from an Inter-Disciplinary Team Perspective

The preceding examples and case studies outline examples of goal statements specific to therapeutic recreation. These case studies (p. 110-120) and tables (10-14) should be studied, and case studies 3 through 6 may be completed for practice. Case Study 7 (p. 122) illustrates goal setting from an inter-disciplinary team setting and emphasizes the opportunity for collaboration among team members to maximize goal achievement and facilitate optimal client functioning.

This is the typical type of process encountered in rehabilitation settings. The case attempts to illustrate how the assessment of the client is multi-disciplinary and how goal setting is an inter-disciplinary, interactive process requiring input from all team members. It also shows how each team member's activities are targeted towards achieving the goal and how the therapeutic recreation professional contributes to this process using the LCM. It will be realized that there is a large measure of pragmatism in choosing goals and defining them. The emphasis in a busy program is on getting the job done. Without goal setting it would be difficult for everyone to know where they are going and what they are trying to achieve; but goal setting cannot become an end in itself as can happen if the team becomes overly concerned about what is a goal and what is an objective, etc. The ultimate test is whether or not the client's needs are being met.

Although illustrated by a client in rehabilitation, this process, with modification, can be employed in long-term care settings and in the community when several therapists are involved in the care of a client.

Linking the LCM with Goal Setting

The previous example (Case Study 7) suggested the use of the LCM to help guide and monitor the client's progress towards the goal. We will now examine use of the LCM in goal setting in more detail. The concept is fairly simple and depends upon the ability to express the goal in the same terms used to assess the client. Thus, for example, Albert may upon admission, score 3 on the Community Integration Skills subscale. One then asks what level of independent function is needed to achieve the goal. It might be decided that a score of 6 is needed. This then becomes the target for the specific intervention designed to improve community integration skills. Conversely in long-term care settings, rather than expecting significant improvement in client functioning to meet the challenges of an activity and assuming limited potential for such improvement, it will be the planned activity or program which will have to be tailored to accommodate the client's abilities and limitations.

A goal implies a certain future level of achievement to be aimed for. Goals can, however, be expressed in terms of the LCM scores required to meet them. Targets can then be set for the overall LCM, or for

Case Study 7

Albert is 79 years old. Over the past year he has experienced a deterioration in his health. He began to experience chest pain on exercise a year ago and was diagnosed as having angina. This rapidly deteriorated over the following weeks and he was admitted to hospital with constant chest pain. Albert eventually went for urgent cardiac surgery to have coronary artery bypass grafting. Although the operation went well he was slow to recover from the anesthetic. Albert spent 10 days in the intensive care unit during which time he developed pneumonia. It took a further 3 weeks for him to recover to the point where care in the acute care hospital was no longer needed. Albert was too weak to return directly home and went to the rehabilitation unit. Unfortunately 2 days after admission he fell and fractured his right hip. After further surgery in the acute care hospital, Albert returned quickly to the rehabilitation unit.

Previous Functioning: Prior to his illness, Albert was very well and independent. He lives with his wife in a one floor home with 6 steps at the front door and 4 steps at the back. His previous interests were reading, going regularly to the theatre and bowling. Albert and his wife liked shopping together and frequently went walking, outside in the summer, and in the shopping mall during the winter. Albert clearly expresses his desire to get home as soon as possible.

Assessment at this Point Revealed:

- Albert has lost 20 lbs. in weight
- there is evidence of some confusion (it was felt his pain medication (codeine) might be contributing to this)
- Albert has an indwelling urinary catheter
- there is clear deconditioning with proximal muscle weakness
- Albert needs help getting out of a chair, as well as in and out of bed
- Albert can walk a few steps with a walker and one assistant; is limited by weakness and pain
- Albert easily becomes short of breath which could partly be deconditioning and partly compromised cardiac function
- there is some limitation of hip flexion on the fractured side such that sitting up comfortably is difficult
- Albert's leisure involvement ceased at the onset of his illness

The physiotherapist feels that she can improve Albert's proximal muscle strength and his mobility. She would like his pain to be better controlled and the urinary catheter to be removed. The physiotherapist feels Albert would do better if his memory improved. The physician and nursing staff undertake to remove the catheter and manage the subsequent bladder function (they establish their own goals around Albert's bladder and subsequent continence management, realizing, in turn, that if he is mobile enough to get to the washroom himself it will be much easier). The physician will stop the codeine and substitute acetaminophen in the hope that the confusion will improve. The nutritionist will address the weight loss.

The physiotherapist might formulate the following goal:

Goal Statement: Albert will walk 200 feet independently with the use of a straight cane within the next 2-3 weeks.

This goal has the advantage that (1) it is a measurable change in function (and will be detected by, for example, a change in FIM score), and (2) it is achievable within his expected length of stay in the unit (3 weeks). However, this goal has the disadvantage that, in its isolation and narrowness, it might not be sufficient to meet Albert's mobility needs. For example, if the distance from the parking lot to the theatre is 300 feet, then Albert will have to give up one source of significant pleasure. Alternatively, the team can establish, in collaboration with Albert and his wife, a more complex goal:

Goal Statement: Albert will return to his previous lifestyle by the time he is discharged.

This goal is too nonspecific. It might also be unrealistic for Albert's present admission as a full functional recovery might take several months and a totally unmodified lifestyle might not be possible. A better goal is:

Goal Statement: Upon return home (discharge) Albert will be independent in his personal care, accessing and leaving the home, and will be able to attend the theatre and go shopping with his wife. Prior to discharge Albert's potential for returning to bowling will be assessed, although it is expected this will be a longer term goal which could be addressed if he attends the Day Hospital after discharge.

This "goal statement", it will be realized, actually contains several goals which could, if so desired, be written as a list of distinct goals, and each goal linked with a list of sub-goals. As an exercise the reader could list these separate goals and then list the functions that would be needed to achieve each goal.

With this goal statement specific subgoals or tasks can be identified as components of this particular challenge. In order to achieve this goal, Albert will for example (with possible team members who might choose to address these sub-goals):

- need to walk at least 300 feet independently with or without an aid (physiotherapy; nursing; therapeutic recreation)
- get in and out of a car (physiotherapy; therapeutic recreation)
- manage the steps into his house; will a railing be required? (physiotherapy; occupational therapy)
- be continent of urine; if, for example, Albert is on a diuretic following his heart surgery it might be possible and safe for him to take the diuretic after he returns home from shopping rather than before setting out (physician; nursing)
- be able to toilet independently (nursing; occupational therapy; physiotherapy)
- be able to sit for 1-2 hours without discomfort (nursing; physiotherapy)
- be able to concentrate on the theatre performance and follow the plot; his confusion will need to be assessed and monitored as his medication is altered and time passes (physician; therapeutic recreation; other therapies)

The occupational therapist may wish to do a home visit and the therapeutic recreation specialist will probably want to take Albert to visit the theatre and bowling alley, or at the very least evaluate Albert's abilities in the hospital's programs. The LCM will provide insight into Albert's ability to make his arrangements, organize himself to get there on time, interact appropriately with others, etc.

Target scores on the LCM subscales can be set to reflect the needs of the subgoals and steps (or strategies or task objectives) can be initiated to reach these subgoals. The progress towards these subgoals can be plotted over Albert's 3 week stay and continued by the therapeutic recreation specialist in the Day Hospital if it is determined that Albert would benefit from going there. This approach identifies:

- a major goal for the client, family and team to aim for
- discipline specific and interdisciplinary sub-goals which are component parts of the primary goal
- underlying specific target scores (LCM) which help the TRS monitor progress towards the mutually agreed upon primary goal

Regular team meetings will track Albert's progress, discuss problems and review the feasibility of the goal. The success of the program can be expressed as:

① the "change scores" on the FIM,[7] LCM or other more specific scales (e.g., Mini-Mental State Examination (MMSE);[8] Berg Balance Scale;[9] etc.)

② the achievement or non-achievement of the subgoals

③ the achievement or non-achievement of the overall goal

④ the degrees of achievement of the subgoals or overall goal, if goal achievement scaling is employed (see p. 132)

Full and accurate charting is essential not only for communication among team members but in some instances for payment purposes.

The following table provides examples of possible measurable sub-goals and strategies for Albert, which disciplines might have primary responsibility for these goals, and also which disciplines might be well suited to collaborate on these sub-goals to help maximize Albert's performance in these areas.

TABLE 15. EXAMPLES OF HEALTH PROFESSIONALS COLLABORATING IN THE DEVELPOPMENT OF CLIENT (SUB)GOALS AND STRATEGIES

(SUB) GOALS	STRATEGIES	PRIMARY RESPONSIBILITY	POTENTIAL FOR COLLABORATION WITH . . .
1. Albert will walk 300 feet independently and safely, with a cane by discharge.	In order to achieve this: i) he will attend physiotherapy daily, for 45 minutes, in order to improve his balance, work on muscle strength, hip flexion and improve tolerance. ii) Albert will require a walker initially but is expected to progress to a cane before discharge in 3 weeks. iii) an assessment of car transfers will be done several days before discharge. iv) ability to ascend and descend stairs will be assessed as mobility and balance improve. v) muscle strength, balance, endurance and distance walked will be monitored daily.	Physiotherapy	① walk 300 feet (Nursing; Therapeutic Recreation) ② car transfer (Therapeutic Recreation) ③ ascend and descend stairs to his home - possible environmental modification (e.g., railing required) (Occupational Therapy)
2. Albert will achieve independence in his ADLs (toileting, bathing and dressing) by discharge.	In order to achieve this: i) Albert will attend occupational therapy daily, for 30 minutes. ii) adaptive aids to help with lower body dressing will be explored with Albert and his wife. iii) a home visit will be scheduled to assess the need for home modifications prior to discharge	Occupational Therapy	① toileting and bathing (Nursing; Physiotherapy)
3. Albert will achieve full control of his bladder function by discharge.	In order to achieve this: i) Albert's catheter will be removed and his urination monitored to detect retention. ii) assessment of post-void residual may be required. Albert will be walked to the toilet regularly. independence in ADLs will be encouraged and monitored daily. iv) cognition will be monitored daily.	Nursing	① removal of catheter and monitoring for urinary retention (Physician)

(Table 15 continued on page 126)

(SUB) GOALS	STRATEGIES	PRIMARY RESPONSIBILITY	POTENTIAL FOR COLLABORATION WITH . . .
4. Albert will demonstrate the ability to independently attend the theatre and go shopping with his wife.	In order to achieve this: i) he will attend therapeutic recreation daily, for 45 minutes in order to improve his sitting tolerance, work on improving his concentration with an activity of personal interest, and to improve his mobility. ii) community outings will be scheduled to the theatre and a local shopping mall to assess Albert's ability to initiate, plan and follow-through on these community interests.	Therapeutic Recreation	① all team members

Although these (sub)goals may fall under the domain of specific disciplines, all interdisciplinary team members will work on them to facilitate optimal functioning in all areas (e.g., therapeutic recreation specialist encouraging mobility; nursing encouraging Albert's ADL independence , etc.)

specific LCM subscales if only one or two areas are seen to be problematic. For example, with a spinal cord injury leisure skills may be of particular importance rather than, say, interpersonal skills which are less likely to have been adversely affected by the injury. It is in keeping with current thinking that goals be more than gains in function, but represent improvement in areas such as quality of life, life satisfaction, etc. Such goals are more client-driven but, however idiosyncratic, they can be broken down into specific functional abilities, which in turn can be expressed by the subscales of the LCM. Thus a certain score on the leisure awareness, leisure attitude, leisure skills and social contact subscales may be felt to be necessary to meet the goal. The goal can be expressed as an LCM profile and a total LCM score which then become the targets for the therapeutic recreation professional. The final level of function achieved should equal this score, and, if so, the goal has been perfectly achieved. The degree to which the goal has been achieved can be expressed as, for example, the final score as a percentage of the target or goal score. If there is a functional shortfall this will be less than 100%, if there have been greater gains than expected, it will exceed 100%. One potential problem is that the required final total score may be reached if there is over achievement in one area, and underachievement in another. If this latter was critical to goal achievement the goal would not be reached although the required total score was. In practice, however, this is not usually a significant problem but is one potential pitfall of this approach.

We can again, here, touch on how we view a problem. Albert's "limitations" can be defined in terms of his medical diseases (ischaemic heart disease, fractured hip) but this, though legitimate, is of limited help to the team. These problems could be expressed in terms of the functional deficits so produced which is, in fact, the role of the assessment. One will soon realize that expressing deficits as problems has its limitations. What, for example, does one do with a deficit that is irrelevant to the achievement of the goal? Is it really a problem? We have found that it is of more practical value to define problems as the degree to which a particular function falls short of the level required to achieve the goal. In the above rehabilitation example, for instance, the problem is how to move Albert from a score of 3 on the Community Integration Skills subscale to a score of 6. If we fail, the goal will not be achieved.

Case Study 2 (p. 129) illustrates how to set goals once the therapeutic recreation assessment has been completed, and scores assigned to the LCM subscales. In this case (Case Study 2), Anthony is a 37 year old male who sustained a severe brain injury in a motorcycle accident. Anthony's family is overwhelmed by his injury. They know nothing about brain injury and have no idea what to expect as Anthony begins the process of rehabilitation. Anthony has problems with judgement, self-care and community living skills, as well as problems with balance and mobility (see Case Study 2 for more detail). Upon completion of the assessment, the therapeutic recreation specialist determines that Anthony is at the following functional levels:

Leisure Awareness	3
Leisure Attitude	2
Leisure Skills	3
Cultural/Social Behaviours	1
Interpersonal Skills	2
Community Integration Skills	2
Social Contact	4
Community Participation	2

Anthony's expected length of stay on the unit is 4 weeks. It is anticipated that he will then be discharged to his parent's home.

By a process of interaction with the family and Anthony, goals must be set. This is not simple and requires an element of education of the family and client about the injury and its prognosis. The family and Anthony will express their hopes, and the therapeutic recreation professional and interdisciplinary team can offer an opinion on the client's likely level of independence, which might reveal that the hopes are unrealistic. Through a process akin to negotiation a goal will be set, which includes much that seems worthwhile to the client and family while being realistic. The degree of progress to be expected toward that goal during Anthony's stay will be outlined. This process might not be simple and indeed might evolve over a period of time as Anthony and his family adjust to the problem and its future implications. The therapeutic recreation professional must now determine where to target her intervention by identifying those areas of functioning that have the greatest negative impact on Anthony's life. The therapeutic recreation professional must keep in mind that while there are many areas related to leisure functioning that she might work on with Anthony, she only has 4 weeks before his expected discharge. It is therefore critical that she exercise her skill as a professional.

With increasing pressure to shorten lengths of stay it has become increasingly important for the system as a whole to function in a co-ordinated fashion, offering a continuum of care to the client. It is common for each segment of the system to receive the client from elsewhere (e.g., acute care hospital) and subsequently pass him or her along to the next segment (e.g., community care or long-term care). Good communication between segments is critical and it is important that the client's overall goals don't become compartmentalized, but provide guidance for each segment of the system as the client moves through. Each segment moves the client a certain distance towards the final goal.

It is legitimate for a segment, for example rehabilitation, to set sub-goals for the relatively short stay, provided those sub-goals contribute to the achievement of the larger goal. Under these circumstances the therapeutic recreation specialist might be obliged to work to bring about partial progress toward the goals, focusing specifically on the areas where the most important gains can be made in the given time.

Thus, in this example the therapeutic recreation professional might feel that, in the 4 weeks available, she should focus on Anthony's social behaviours and interpersonal skills, as these are the areas most likely to limit overall progress toward the final goal of getting Anthony home, and capable of meaningful interaction with his family and friends. These particular skills are also necessary antecedents for community integration, the development of social networks, and ultimately maximizing community participation.

FIGURE 34. EXAMPLES OF POSSIBLE GOALS FOR ANTHONY

LCM Subscales:

Cultural/ Social Behaviours

Within 3-4 weeks (or by discharge) Anthony will, with cueing, demonstrate socially acceptable manners, with approprpiate dress and cleanliness, and be tolerant of others in small group situations of 6-8 clients. (LCM score 4)

Interpersonal Skills

Within 3-4 weeks (or by discharge) Anthony will demonstrate the ability to participate in a task of personal interest for a minimum of 15 minutes, in a small group situation of 6-8 clients. (LCM score 4)

Note: These goals are seen as being of primary importance for Anthony as without these basic skills further progress related to therapeutic recreation intervention will be seriously compromised, and the more global, long-term goals of increasing Anthony's social contacts and his participation in the community cannot be achieved. The therapeutic recreation professional therefore identifies these as critical areas of focus for Anthony's limited length of stay in her program.

Case Study 2

Anthony is a 37 year old male who sustained a severe brain injury in a motorcycle race. Prior to his accident he held an international ranking and devoted much of his time to racing. He worked occasionally as a plumber to supplement his income. Shortly after his accident his girlfriend terminated their relationship.

Anthony now requires medication to control his excitability and is somewhat rigid in his thinking. He experiences pain in his lower back which causes agitation. In the past, much of Anthony's time was spend socializing and drinking after motorcycle races. The only activities of interest to him at present are motorcycle racing and watching television. He has unrealistic expectations about being able to race again and is unable to identify why it might be important for him to be involved in other activities. Anthony requires assistance to participate in facility programs and often if in a program, requires constant re-direction by his therapist to maintain his involvement. He does not self-initiate, often lacks the ability to focus, his judgement is impaired and at times he is at risk for his own safety. While Anthony does not participate for long in group settings, he does interact on an individual level with his therapist and with family members. He interacts reasonably well with those he knows; his interaction with others is often inappropriate in that he talks excessively, tends to confabulate and is socially disinhibited. In group situations Anthony is often intolerant of others and at times has become verbally and physically aggressive. Anthony requires physical intervention in regard to his manners and to dress appropriately for the weather; he often resists the assistance provided by his therapist. He requires assistance from his therapist to plan and follow through on outings to the community, and often these outings have to be cut short due to Anthony's fatigue and/or behaviour. Anthony, at this point, does not participate in community programs, spends most of his time watching television in his room, and only takes part in facility programs with direct assistance from his therapist.

FUNCTIONAL INDICATORS	ADM __/__/__ dd mth yr	__/__/__ dd mth yr	__/__/__ dd mth yr	__/__/__ dd mth yr	D/C __/__/__ dd mth yr	F/U __/__/__ dd mth yr
LEISURE AWARENESS	3					
LEISURE ATTITUDE	2					
LEISURE SKILLS	3					
CULTURAL/SOCIAL BEHAVIOURS	1					
INTERPERSONAL SKILLS	2					
COMMUNITY INTEGRATION SKILLS	2					
SOCIAL CONTACT	4					
COMMUNITY PARTICIPATION	2					
TOTAL LCM SCORE (out of 56) -ADMISSION	19 / 56	DISCHARGE/FOLLOW-UP			/ 56	/ 56

ADM = ADMISSION/BASELINE D/C = DISCHARGE F/U = FOLLOW-UP (≥ 2 MONTHS)

Note: Enter a value for each Functional Indicator
Enter "0" for "not assess

The LCM and Change/Gain Scores

A specific statement of the functional improvement, of a client, achieved over time (and resulting from defined intervention) provides a measure of outcome. The difference in score from baseline (admission or start of program) to time of plateau of score, discharge or other meaningful point, is the change or gain score. Change in total LCM score sums the overall gain in client functioning related to leisure.

It is possible, based on client assessment, experience, and knowledge of the prognosis of the disease or injury, to predict the degree of improvement that could be expected by Anthony over a defined period of time. The therapeutic recreation professional might then say "I think I can get this type of client to score 6 on the Social Interaction subscale", for example. The goal then is a certain gain in score on a particular subscale. Even if that score is not reached (e.g., this particular client only reached a score of 5) there will likely be some improvement which can be expressed as a gain score and provide some positive outcome for the client and program. If one chooses to measure gain scores (degree of improvement) rather than the achievement of goals, there are certain precautions to bear in mind if gain scores are subsequently used to evaluate the programs. This requires the pooling of data from many individuals that have passed through the program. Some of these concerns have been touched on already, and are covered fully in the paper by Johnson, Keith and Hinderer.[6] In brief, however, the scale measuring the gain must have approximately equal intervals if one wants to combine gain scores across different individuals. The scale must have good test-retest reliability and be measuring a function that is fairly stable on a day-to-day basis. If the function or behaviour being measured shows wide fluctuation from day to day (e.g., client is socially appropiate one day, quite inappropriate the next), these fluctuations can swamp any true change over time, or, even more problematic, be misleadingly attributed to intervention. Thus apparent improvement over the course of intervention might simply reflect randomly poor performance at admission and fortuitously good performance at the time of discharge re-assessment. Two or more measurements at admission and discharge might be needed to overcome this difficulty. Johnston, Keith and Hinderer[6] discuss some of the statistical safeguards to observe if the combining of gain scores is to be done and the reader is referred to their paper for fuller discussion.

When measuring outcomes (change or gain in client function) it is important that therapeutic recreation professionals: (1) identify and choose a client behaviour or function that is expected to change with therapeutic recreation intervention; (2) choose a psychometrically sound (standardized) instrument that is sensitive to change, to measure the client behaviour or function of interest (see Chapter 1); (3) determine time intervals for repeat administration of the instrument; and (4) collect data and analyze the results of the information collected.

The LCM is a standardized tool that provides therapeutic recreation professionals with a method to measure client outcomes related to leisure functioning and therapeutic recreation intervention. By using the LCM to: (1) summarize information related to client functioning gathered through a comprehensive therapeutic recreation assessment process; (2) identify priority areas for intervention; (3) guide therapeutic recreation intervention; and (4) by completing the LCM again upon program completion, client discharge or at other pre-determined time intervals, therapeutic recreation professionals are able to monitor change or gain in client functioning.

Goal Attainment Scaling and Therapeutic Recreation Practice

An alternative approach is to use goal attainment scaling methodology.[1,2,3,4,5] As mentioned in Chapter 1, this is a method for measuring the *degree* of goal achievement, which creates an individualized 5-point scale (-2,-1,0,+1, +2) of potential outcomes for each client (see Figure 35).

Goal attainment scaling is a feasible and practical way to identify, set and monitor realistic, observable client goals. Goal attainment scaling personalizes client goals yet permits comparison of goal achievement among clients, is suited for both discipline-specific and inter-disciplinary team use, and allows scores for each of the client's goals to be statistically combined into an overall numerical score. Setting meaningful therapeutic recreation goals (whether using the LCM, goal attainment scaling or a combination of both approaches) takes professional skill and practice. Just as with using the LCM, therapeutic recreation practitioners using the goal attainment scaling method to develop and scale goals for their clients should have substantial training in therapeutic recreation procedures to ensure that meaningful therapeutic recreation goals are set and the level of goal achievement is accurately determined.

Goal attainment scaling requires therapeutic recreation professionals to: (1) identify limitations in client behaviour or functioning that can be improved through intervention and that are expected to change; (2) determine what outcomes related to the behaviour or functioning of interest will identify change resulting from therapeutic recreation intervention; (3) determine the 5 levels of change, beginning with the realistic, expected outcome (midpoint) being sure to take into consideration factors such as the client's anticipated length of stay, discharge prognosis, etc. and then determining the most and least likely levels; and (4) defining time intervals for monitoring and measuring goal achievement (see Figures 36 & 38). It is generally recommended that a minimum of 3 and up to 5 goals are developed and scaled. Once the goal levels have been identified, the therapeutic recreation practitioner should "mark" the current level of functioning of the client (see Figures 36 & 38). Goal levels achieved are again marked (with a different symbol) following completion of the intervention, program or at pre-determined time lines.

When developing goal levels, therapeutic recreation professionals should take care to be specific and clear in their goals, avoid overlapping, or leaving functional gaps between goals from one level to the next to ensure accurate scoring, focus on a single behaviour or function at each level (or alternatively if addressing more than one behaviour or function at the same level, avoid simultaneous change, rather stagger the expected change in behaviours or functioning), and if possible do not leave any of the levels (-2 to +2) blank[4].

Goal attainment scaling may be done in two different ways, with varying degrees of sophistication. Firstly, at the simplest level, goals are "unweighted" (all considered of equal importance) and the therapeutic recreation professional (or inter-disciplinary team) upon completion of the intervention or program (or at pre-determined intervals along the way) simply states whether the goals have been met, exceeded or were underachieved, by examining initial and final goal levels. For example, Figure 36 illustrates that the client for whom these particular goals were set (13 year old adolescent) achieved or exceeded all of the goals that were set. Following completion of a comprehensive assessment and discussion with the client and her family, for example, it was mutually determined that lack of awareness of recreation resources, the leisure attitude of the client's family and the client's social skills were important areas of concern that could be targeted for intervention. Once the expected outcomes or program goals have been established (taking into consideration factors such as the client's

FIGURE 35. GOAL SETTING AND ACHIEVEMENT FORM

NAME: ______________________ DATE: ______________

GOAL ATTAINMENT LEVELS	GOAL AREAS				
Much less than expected -2					
Somewhat less than expected -1					
Expected level (Program Goal) 0					
Somewhat better than expected +1					
Much better than expected +2					
Comments					

FIGURE 36. SETTING THERAPEUTIC RECREATION GOALS USING GOAL ATTAINMENT SCALING

NAME:______________________________ **DATE:** ____________________

GOAL ATTAINMENT LEVELS	GOAL AREAS			
	Awareness of Resources	*Leisure Attitude (Family)*	*Social Skills*	
Much less than expected -2	*No knowledge or utilization of agency or community resources; open to information though* ✔	*Belief that child will never be able to participate in recreation programs; protective environment only*	*Interacts on a 1:1 only with family or TRS* ✔	
Somewhat less than expected -1	*Initiate involvement in specialized agency programs only; protective environment necessary*	*Belief child can participate in agency and specialized community programs offered in partnership with the agency* ✔	*Interacts on a 1:1 with family, TRS and others (strangers)*	
Expected level (Program Goal) 0	*Knowledge and utilization of specialized community recreation programs* ✱	*Belief that child can participate in specialized and some general community* ✱ *programs (e.g. YMCA)*	*Participates in a short term task in the presence of others (group situation)*	
Somewhat better than expected +1	*Knowledge and utilization of specialized and at least one general community program;*	*Belief that child can fully participate in specialized and general community programs of interest*	*Begins to respect the rights of others, shares, co-operates, etc.* ✱	
Much better than expected +2	*Knowledge and involvement in a variety of general community recreation programs*	*Belief that child can fully participate, and be competent in, general community programs of interest*	*Independent and appropriate participation in individual and group situations*	
Comments				

✔ = baseline rating of client/family ability
✱ = rating of client/family ability at time of program completion

anticipated length of stay, discharge prognosis, etc.) and subsequent goal levels have been developed (ranging from better than expected/less than expected (+1 & -1) to the most/least likely (+2 & -2) goals to be achieved), the therapeutic recreation professional "marks" the client's *current* level of functioning. In this case check marks were used to identify the client's current level of functioning. Upon completion of the intervention or program (or at other pre-determined time intervals) the client's progress is reviewed and achievement of goals is evaluated. The therapeutic recreation professional then "marks" the level that best describes the client's level of functioning at this point in time. In this case an asterisk was used to differentiate the client's current level of functioning from their initial level of functioning (check marks). It can then be quickly and easily seen whether or not the client has achieved the expected level of outcomes.

Secondly, if desired, goals may also be "weighted" or prioritized in terms of importance. It is generally recommended that goals are not weighted unless it is clinically relevant. There are other factors to think about if one is considering weighting the goals. For example, weighting goals at the inter-disciplinary team level can be both problematic or potentially disruptive, as well as time consuming. If the team decides to identify goals that are more important than others (prioritize goals), it is not uncommon for lengthy debates to follow. This process can be disruptive to fostering inter-disciplinary team collaboration and therefore is best avoided. However, on the other hand, weighting may be helpful if weighting criteria can be agreed upon by the inter-disciplinary team. For example if a situation is considered critical certain interventions may be required before others. Or, if it is determined that unless a specific goal is achieved, the remaining goals are compromised it may be helpful to "order" goals logically. Another alternative to weighting might be for the inter-disciplinary team to mutually collaborate on the goals, along with the client and their family and then abdicate, letting the client and family determine those areas most important to them (promoting continued and active involvement by the client and their family). Goal attainment scaling from a discipline-specific perspective is more suited to "weighting" than from an inter-disciplinary team perspective, for the reasons outlined above. Therapeutic recreation professionals might find it helpful to prioritize goals with their clients, based on their professional judgment and experience. For example, intuitively it makes sense for a client to develop and maximize leisure skills or social interaction skills *before* establishing goals for community participation.

Goals, developed and scaled, may also be combined and numerically scored. Each client's goals can be amalgamated into a summary score, so that each client ends up with only one number. The goal attainment formula or score:

$$= 50 + \frac{10\Sigma(w_i x_i)}{\sqrt{(.7\Sigma w_i^2 + .3(\Sigma w_i)^2)}}$$

with w_i representing the weighting given to the $_i$th goal, and x_i representing the level or numerical score (-2, -1, 0, +1, +2) of the $_i$th goal (a score of 50 signifies achievement of program goals and an outcome at the expected level). In words, the formula indicates that for each goal the score (-2 to +2) is multiplied by the weighting (use 1 if no weighting is assigned) and then the results for each goal are summed and multiplied by 10. On the bottom line the weightings are squared and then added up, and multiplied by .7. This is added to the sum of all the weightings squared, multiplied by .3. The square root of this final number is taken. This is divided into the upper number (see Figure 37). Initial levels of client functioning, as well the degree of goal achievement by the client, may then be calculated. Conversion tables are available[4,5] for unweighted goals to allow therapeutic recreation professionals to quickly find the same results without having to spend the time working through the goal attainment formula.

FIGURE 37. CALCULATING THE GOAL ATTAINMENT SCORE FOR THE EXAMPLE PROVIDED IN FIGURE 36.

In the example given (Figure 36), where no weightings are applied (w = 1) the formula yields the following result for

Baseline Scores:

$$= 50 + \frac{10 \text{ x } (1 \text{ x } -2 + 1 \text{ x } -1 + 1 \text{ x } -2)}{\sqrt{.7(1^2 + 1^2 + 1^2) + .3(1 + 1 + 1)^2}}$$

$$= 50 + \frac{10 \text{ x } -5}{\sqrt{.7 \text{ x } 3 + .3 \text{ x } 9}}$$

$$= 50 + \frac{-50}{\sqrt{2.1 + 2.7}}$$

$$= 50 + \frac{-50}{\sqrt{4.8}}$$

$$= 50 + \frac{-50}{\sqrt{2.19}}$$

$$= 50 - 22.83$$

$$= 27.17$$

Final Scores:

$$= 50 + \frac{10 \text{ x } (1 \text{ x } 0 + 1 \text{ x } 0 + 1 \text{ x } 1)}{\sqrt{.7 \text{ x } 3 + .3 \text{ x } 9}}$$

$$= 50 + \frac{10}{\sqrt{4.8}}$$

$$= 50 + 4.57$$

$$= 54.57$$

Therefore this client's score has improved from 27.17 to 54.57. The 10 on the top line is there simply to avoid having to use small numbers and the addition of 50 is for the convenience of avoiding negative numbers. This is sometimes referred to as the T score, which relates to a population defined as having a mean of 50 (rather than 0) and a standard deviation of 10 (rather than 1). It will be realized that if the goals are perfectly attained (i.e., all final scores = 0), the final total score will be 50. The client in this example, therefore, did slightly better than expected.

Figure 38 illustrates goal setting and evaluation of client goal achievement from an inter-disciplinary team perspective. As can be seen, a variety of goals have been developed and scaled for this particular client (Anthony, Case Study 2) with input from all inter-disciplinary team members, including therapeutic recreation. In this particular case, all of the program goals and expected outcomes have either been met or exceeded. For practice the reader can calculate the baseline and final scores for Anthony from Figure 38 using the formula and process indicated above. The scores are respectively, 22.86 and 53.02.

While the goal areas clearly fall under the domains of specific professional disciplines, for example, social skills clearly falls under the professional domain of therapeutic recreation, balance and mobility under physiotherapy, problem solving related to homemaking and community living under occupational therapy, etc., this approach promotes collaboration among the various inter-disciplinary team members. For example, therapeutic recreation professionals aware of balance, family education and community living goals can assist in optimizing client and family functioning in these areas by collaborating with other health professionals around these areas and incorporating appropriate strategies for these areas into the therapeutic recreation intervention provided. Likewise, other health professionals can consult with the therapeutic recreation professional around the issues of social interaction and the client's social skills and help maximize client functioning by reinforcing therapeutic recreation intervention strategies in their involvement with the client, if appropriate.

The goal attainment scaling method is somewhat relative in that the goal can be very specific for the client, and the under and over achieved levels can be similarly unique to the client. Thus, mobility goals for one client may be quite different than for another, and the intervals on the scale between the 5 levels defined for each client may be quite different. In practice, however, clients of a similar type tend to have similar functional limitations and are expected to achieve similar goals. Thus there is much less diversification in the goals than might at first sight seem likely. When evaluating goal achievement and recording these levels of achievement, care should be taken to remain objective and not to bias the scoring in an attempt to improve the apparent success of the program. Also, one of the cautions regarding the goal attainment scaling method is that the goal attainment scaling format does not include a mechanism for monitoring or ensuring feedback regarding client progress toward goals set. It is therefore important that the therapeutic recreation professional, upon completing the goal setting process, determine time intervals for follow-up to examine client goal achievement.

This section on goal attainment scaling was included to simply highlight this method as an alternative to measuring client outcomes and to make therapeutic recreation professionals aware of this option. There are many excellent references detailing goal attainment scaling methods, validity and reliability information, as well as scoring procedures. Books and papers professionals might find particularly helpful include: (1) *Goal Attainment Scaling: Application, Theory and Measurement* by Kiresuk, Smith & Cardillo;[4] (2) *The Use of Goal Attainment Scaling in a Geriatric Care Setting* by Stolee, Rockwood, Fox & Streiner;[2] and (3) *Goal Attainment Scaling* by Kiresuk & Lund.[5]

Both procedures, change/gain scores and goal attainment scaling, as well as a combination of these approaches provide therapeutic recreation professionals with options for measuring outcomes related to therapeutic recreation intervention.

FIGURE 38. GOAL ATTAINMENT SCALING FROM AN INTER-DISCIPLINARY TEAM PERSPECTIVE

NAME:____________________ **DATE:** ______________

GOAL ATTAINMENT LEVELS	GOAL AREAS				
	Balance	*Mobility*	*Family Education re: injury*	*Social Skills*	*Judgement/ Problem Solving*
Much less than expected -2	*Unable to walk outdoors or on uneven surfaces. Unable to ascend/descend a flight of stairs.* ✔	*Unable to transfer - assist x2. Dependent bed mobility.* ✔	*No understanding or information re: son's injury.* ✔	*Interacts 1:1 only with family or his therapist.*	*Unable to perform homemaking/ community living skills(e.g., meal prep.; grocery shopping; laundry; money management; etc.)* ✔
Somewhat less than expected -1	*Able to walk outdoors on uneven surfaces, ascend/descend flight of stairs with assistance.*	*1 person assist with transfers from bed to w/c; w/c to toilet. Independent in bed mobility with use of trapeze.*	*Client and family have limited understanding or information re: injury.*	*Interacts on a 1:1 with family, therapist and others (strangers).* ✔	*Able to prepare meals with assistance; laundry with assistance.*
Expected level (Program Goal) 0	*Able to walk outdoors on uneven surfaces; ascend/descend 1 flight of stairs.* ✱	*Independent transfer, with standby assistance, from bed-w/c; w/c to toilet; independent in bed mobility without use of trapeze).*	*Client and family have understanding and knowledge of brain injury and its sequelae.* ✱	*Participates in a short term task in the presence of others (group situation).* ✱	*Prepares* ✱ *meals/laundry safely & independently; grocery shopping with assistance; money management tasks with assistance.*
Somewhat better than expected +1	*Able to walk outdoors on uneven surfaces but limited by time and distance; ascend/descend stairs*	*Independent transfer from bed-w/c; w/c to toilet; independent bed mobility.* ✱	*Client and family have understanding and knowledge of brain injury and its sequelae, and share this knowledge with others.*	*Begins to respect the rights of others, shares, co-operates, etc.*	*Independent in meal/preparation, grocery shopping and laundry. Money management with assistance.*
Much better than expected +2	*Independent with community ambulation (not limited by time and distance)*	*Ability to transfer independently in a variety of situations. Independent in bed mobility.*		*Independent and appropriate participation in individual and group situations*	*Independent in homemaking community living skills (e.g., meal prep.; grocery shopping; laundry; money management.*
Comments					

✔ = baseline rating of client/family ability
✱ = rating of client/family ability at time of program completion

Blending LCM Scores with Goal Attainment Scaling Methods

The two approaches to measuring outcomes (change and gain scores using a standardized instrument or goal attainment scaling) are not mutually exclusive and can be blended. For example, the LCM subscales can be used to define the levels that make up the 5-point goal attainment scale, such that the 5 levels correspond to sequential scores on the LCM. The levels on the LCM subscales are described in generic terms and the therapeutic recreation specialist must exercise professional judgement in applying the scale to individual clients. The goal attainment scaling method can, in fact, be used to do just that. The descriptors written for each goal attainment scaling level can represent the personalization of one of the generic levels of the LCM. In this way the goal attainment scaling method becomes a way of operationalizing the LCM for individual clients.

The LCM, by itself, can be used to assess the degree of goal achievement. This can be done in two ways:

① To display the client's success, the degree to which he has reached his goal would be the appropriate expression. Thus, if to achieve his goal a total LCM score of 50 is need but only 40 is reached, he has achieved 80% of his goal.

② To display the program's success a different expression is needed. If the client's baseline score is 30, the program cannot take credit for this. The problem the program was required to solve was to move the client from 30 to 50. As he only reached 40, the program only achieved its goal by 50%.

As mentioned before, many programs or units are part of a continuum of care (particularly those units with very short lengths of stay) and therefore it is not necessary to achieve total success in all goals. The therapeutic recreation professional can decide what contribution his/her program can make, with the expectation that subsequent programs in the continuum of care will take the client further. Thus the therapeutic recreation professional might have decided that although a final score of 50 is to be aimed for, in the time available the client can only be expected to reach a score of 40. This will put a very different complexion on the above calculation and show the program in a much better light. This emphasizes, again, the importance of taking into account the time frame of the program's intervention when setting expectations for the client and the therapeutic recreation specialist.

Can the LCM be used for Continuous Quality Improvement (CQI) Monitoring?

The process of continuous quality improvement (CQI) or total quality management (TQM) implies performance, evaluation of performance and feedback of the evaluation to permit program modifications in the hope that outcome will improve. The LCM, coupled with goal setting can provide that feedback. This is illustrated in Figure 39. The percentage of goals met indicates the number of times a goal score set under a particular category (subscale) was actually achieved. For example, under leisure skills, although the average score in the 8 clients increased from 3.8 to 6.6, only 7 (87%) of the clients actually reached their target. In this particular department (Kernan Hospital, TR Department, Maryland, U.S.A.) achievement of 80% of goals set is considered satisfactory. A shortfall, as occurred in the Leisure Attitude subscale, prompts further analysis to determine why. This process, of course, requires insight into the therapeutic process and what interventions are expected to achieve what outcomes and hence, which interventions require improvement. An alternative explanation is, of course, that the therapeutic recreation specialists are setting their goals too high. If this is the case, appropriate education should correct the problem and allow the program to be seen in a better light. It is important, however, that client goals are not compromised simply to improve the program's apparent performance.

Can the LCM be Used for Program Evaluation?

The LCM can form part of an approach to program evaluation providing, as it does, a measure of client improvement and through the summation of client improvements a measure of program effectiveness. However, program evaluation is a specific and complex function which has multiple facets. This can become apparent from a perusal of Figure 12, which shows the Program Logic Model approach to program evaluation. The development of a program logic model is only one such approach. It permits an analysis of the program and its expected outputs and outcomes, the determination of which is dependant upon a clear understanding of program components, processes and program goals. The LCM can clearly help in this, but is only a small part of the overall process. Readers interested in pursuing this further are referred to the references at the end of this chapter.

Linking Therapeutic Recreation Outcomes to General Health Outcomes

It is important to link therapeutic recreation outcomes to broader and more general health outcomes. This is particularly important when therapeutic recreation professionals are preparing reports for funders, purchasers of health services, and their administrators. For example, broader health outcomes might include such things as a client's reduction in anxiety or stress, increased ability to cope, increased mobility, decreased usage of medication, increased ability to manage chronic pain, decrease in schizophrenic symptoms, or the increased ability to manage substance-related stressors. These are but a few examples specific to therapeutic recreation. Readers wishing more detailed information on a summary of health outcomes specific to therapeutic recreation should consult the American Therapeutic Recreation Association (ATRA)[11] *Summary of Health Outcomes* report and the book *Benefits of Therapeutic Recreation: A Consensus View* by Coyle, Kinney, Riley and Shank.[12]

FIGURE 39. USING THE LCM FOR CONTINUOUS QUALITY IMPROVEMENT MONITORING.

Unit:	Traumatic Brain Injury	Threshold:	Minimum 80%
Diagnosis:	TBI, aneurysms	Number of Clients:	8
		Time Frame:	01 April 92 - 01 June 92

Category	Average Score Admission	Average Score Discharge	Percentage of Goals Met
Leisure Awareness	4.6	6.8	100%
Leisure Attitude	4.8	6.6	75%
Leisure Skills	3.8	6.6	87%
Community Integration Skills	5.5	6.5	87%
Cultural/Social Behaviours	5.0	6.8	100%
Interpersonal Skills	5.1	6.7	87%
Social Contact			
Community Participation			

Number of LCM indicators meeting/exceeding threshold:	5 out of 6
Explanation: Therapists noted early discharges did not allow all goals to be addressed in their entirety.	

Modified By: Linda Hutchinson-Troyer, MGA, CTRS
Patient Therapy Co-ordinator
Brain Injury and Outpatient Therapy Services
Kernan Hospital, Baltimore, Maryland U.S.A.

References

1. Kiresuk, T.J. & Sherman, R.E. (1968). Goal Attainment Scaling: A general method for evaluating comprehensive community mental health programs. Community Mental Health Journal, 4, 443-453.

2. Stolee, P., Rockwood, K., Fox, R.A. & Streiner, D.L. (1992). The use of goal attainment scaling in a geriatric care setting. Journal of the American Geriatrics Society, 40, 574-578.

3. Hartman, D., Borrie, M., Davison, E. & Stolee, P. (1997). Use of goal attainment scaling in a dementia special care unit. American Journal of Alzheimer Disease, 12(3), 111-116.

4. Kiresuk, T.J., Smith, A. & Cardillo, J.E. (1994). Goal attainment scaling: Application, theory and measurement. New Jersey: Lawrence Erlbaum.

5. Kiresuk, T.J. & Lund, S.H. (1978). Goal Attainment Scaling. In C. C. Attkisson, W. A. Hargreaves, M.J. Horowitz & J. E. Sorensen (Eds.), Evaluation of Human Service Programs (pp. 341-370). New York: Academic Press.

6. Johnston, M.V., Keith, R.A. & Hinderer, S.R. (1992). Measurement standards for interdisciplinary medical rehabilitation. Archives of Physical Medicine and Rehabilitation, 73, S-3-S-23.

7. Hamilton, B.B., Granger, F.S., Zielezny, M. & Tashman, J.S. (1987). A uniform national data system for medical rehabilitation. In M.J. Fuhrer (Ed.), Rehabilitation Outcomes: Analysis and Measurement (pp. 137-147). Baltimore: Paul H. Brookes.

8. Yesavage, J.a., Brink, T.L., Rose, T.L., Lum, O., Huang, V., Adey, M. & Leirer, O. (1983). Development and validation of a geriatric depression screening scale: A preliminary report. Journal of Psychiatric Research, 12, 189-204.

9. Berg, K., Wood-Dauphines W. & Williams, J.I. (1995). The Balance Scale: Reliability assessment for elderly residents and patients with an acute stroke. Scandanavian Journal of Rehabilitation Medicine, 27(27)

10. American Therapeutic Recreation Association Summary of health outcomes.

11 Coyle, C.P., Kinney, W.B., Riley, B. & shank, J. W. (Eds.). (1991). Benefits of therapeutic recreation: A consensus view. Pennsylvania: Temple University.

CHAPTER 5

Vision for the Future

SUMMARY

- *Measurement is the basis of science and is the first step toward placing the therapeutic recreation profession on a scientific footing.*
- *There is now a much greater focus on outcome measurement and the determinants of successful outcomes in health care. It is critical that therapeutic recreation professionals begin to demonstrate that successful therapeutic recreation outcomes make a significant contribution to health, and may help to reduce health-related costs.*
- *There is a need for a multi-centred approach to the determination of therapeutic recreation research priorities and the conducting of research projects.*
- *It is critically important that the liaison between practitioners and educators be strenghthened to foster this research.*
- *As a profession we must work together, think creatively, accept the challenge of the present, and ensure our success for the future.*

Chapter 5
Vision for the Future

We have repeatedly made the point throughout this manual, and others are in agreement[1,2,3,4,5,6] that the therapeutic recreation profession needs to be based on a more solid theoretical and scientific footing. The LCM represents a measurement tool based upon a certain approach to therapeutic recreation assessment and intervention, namely leisure education principles. The LCM has undergone rigorous testing to demonstrate its validity and reliability and can form the basis for the measurement of outcomes. Measurement is the basis of science and it is only through measurement and evidence-based information that the value of the profession can be demonstrated in a scientific way.

The purpose of developing the LCM was to make measurement an integral part of daily therapeutic recreation practice. The next step is to use the measurements to demonstrate efficacy. This will need to be done through properly designed studies to demonstrate, for example: (1) improvements in client leisure functioning over time; (2) what produced the improvements; (3) which interventions produce the best results in which client populations and settings; (4) what are the determinants of successful outcomes and the determinants of unsuccessful outcomes; (5) "normative" data for different populations in different settings; (6) standardized approaches to particular interventions; (7) a mechanism of program evaluation to demonstrate program outcomes and compare one program with another; and (8) the demonstration that improvements in leisure functioning brings with it better quaility of life, improved independence and reduced health costs.

There is much to be done, and we hope that the initiative represented by this manual will be a step in the right direction.

A second step in this process will be the development of the international comparative data base. The plan is that an extensive data base can be built by the incorporation of data from many centres, alongside specific descriptors of the programs. This will allow centres to compare their performance with that of other centres with similar characteristics. Once established such a process could form the basis of multi-centred studies designed to put the therapeutic recreation profession on a firm evidence base. More immediately, however, we are aware of the need for therapeutic recreation professionals to demonstrate to their funders, payers and purchasers of health services and administrators their usefulness as a core service. With this in mind we are in the process of developing Windows-based computer software which will provide agencies with a data base for the storage of LCM scores and be capable of producing high impact, visual summary data that may be incorporated into other programs (e.g., Wordperfect; etc.) for reporting purposes. Then for example the therapeutic recreation specialist can show client outcomes or goal achievement for certain client populations, by, for example age and diagnosis, length of stay, etc. as well as simple administrative data (e.g., number of clients seen; length of stay; number of visits; etc.), with a minimum of difficulty and in a readily understandable and report-ready format. This software is in the alpha and beta testing stage and will be available within the next few months. A paediatric version of the LCM is also currently underway. The plans for further development related to the LCM are outlined in Figure 40.

In recent years there has been increased interest in the field of therapeutic recreation, critical appraisal of the profession's contribution and great enthusiasm by therapeutic recreation professionals and educators to move the profession forward. We see a healthy future for the profession provided we are prepared to accept the challenge of demonstrating our worth and evolving into an evidence-based, scientifically founded specialty. This approach must continue to be encouraged by our educational establishments so that our new therapeutic recreation professionals enter the field well versed in the procedures of standardized tool development and utilization, outcome analysis and program evaluation and improvement.

We are most interested in receiving feedback on the manual and the views expressed therein. Please feel free to forward your suggestions and recommendations.

For convenience, we have included a complete copy of the 8 LCM subscales (Appendix A) that may be copied for ease of reference, for intra-agency use. Also included are copies of Case Studies 1 through 6 (Appendix C) that may be copied for practice or training related to the LCM.

FIGURE 40. LCM DEVELOPMENT INITIATIVES CURRENTLY UNDERWAY

MAIN COMPONENTS	LEISURE COMPETENCE MEASURE	PROGRAM EVALUATION	INTERNATIONAL COMPARATIVE DATA BASE
PROCESS	1. To develop an instrument that (a) documents individual change in leisure functioning and (b) guides the development of client-centred measurable goals. 2. To conduct rigorous psychometric testing of the LCM across a variety of settings including: . rehabilitation . geriatric rehabilitation . psychiatry . addiction/chemical dependency . community settings, etc. 3. To develop a paediatric version of the LCM. 4. To develop and publish a User's manual for the LCM. 5. To develop a Windows-based software package for the LCM.	1. To establish a process for evaluating therapeutic recreation delivery systems in order to advocate for necessary changes inservice. 2. To establish a mechanism that documents measures of program function. 3. To conduct goal achievement analysis. 4. To develop and market a software package that will use LCM indicators for continuous quality improvement (CQI) reporting.	1. To establish an international computerized data base that will provide regional, national, international comparative data. 2. To develop a process for training to ensure consistency in definitions and data collection.
OUTPUTS	1. LCM User's Manual and software. 2. Paediatric LCM. 3. Number of facilities involved in LCM testing in (a) Canada and (b) U.S.A. 4. Variety of test sites in (a) Canada and (b) U.S.A. 5. Validity and reliability results.	1. Program evaluation reports using LCM indicators. 2. Number and type of goals achieved. 3. Type of intervention provided. 4. Length of time in program. 5. Change scores. 6. Costs. 7. Dissemination of LCM software.	1. Number of facilities registered with the data base in (a) Canada and (b) U.S.A. 2. Number of client results submitted in (a) Canada and (b) U.S.A. 3. Number of regional and national reports generated.
SHORT-TERM OUTCOMES	1. LCM established as a valid and reliable instrument for measuring outcomes related to leisure functioning. 2. Recognition of the LCM as an outcome instrument by accrediting bodies (e.g. CARF; JCAHO; etc.)	1. Improved accuracy of goal setting. 2. Prediction of rehabilitation potential related to therapeutic recreation intervention and leisure functioning. 3. Evaluation of the efficacy of therapeutic recreation intervention. 4. Increased knowledge of processes, outcomes and costs.	
LONG-TERM OUTCOMES		1. Improved resource utilization. 2. Demonstrated impact of therapeutic recreation on health status. 3. Improved therapeutic recreation service delivery. 4. Standardized and uniform therapeutic recreation service delivery. 5. Therapeutic recreation to be placed on a sound, scientific base.	

RESEARCH

1. To establish a collaborative working group and process for planning and conducting research activities.
2. To identify areas of interest and need for leisure research.
3. To identify and prioritize potential research questions for action.
4. To develop research proposals.
5. To secure research funding.
6. To conduct research activities.
7. To disseminate research findings and their clinical application.
8. To seek to place the therapeutic recreation profession on a firm evidence base.

1. Working group for research.
2. Number of research proposals submitted for funding.
3. Amount of funding secured.
4. Number of studies carried out.
5. Number of papers published.

CONSULTATION/ TRAINING

1. To establish a process for disseminating information on the LCM data system.
2. To conduct formal training sessions outlining the use of the LCM for therapeutic recreation professionals.
3. To develop training packages/ modules for:
   - therapeutic recreation assessment
   - behavioural documentation
   - use of LCM indicators for continuous quality improvement (CQI) monitoring
   - program evaluation
   - usage of the international uniform data system
4. To write a text on outcome measurement for the therapeutic recreation profession.

1. Number of LCM manuals and software disseminated.
2. Number of facilities registered with the LCM data base.
3. Number and type of training sessions provided.
4. Variety of groups requesting training (e.g., practitioners, educators, allied health professionals, etc.)
5. Number of consultations.

References

1. Shank, J.W., Coyle, C.P., Boyd, R. & Kinney, W.B. (196). A classification scheme for therapeutic recreation research grounded in the rehabilitative sciences. Therapeutic Recreation Journal, 30(3), 179-196.

2. Bedini, L. & Wu, Y. (1994). A methodological review of research in *Therapeutic Recreation Journals* from 1986 too 1990. Therapeutic Recreation Journal, 28(2), 87-98.

3. Stumbo, N.J. (1986). A definition of entry-level knowledge for therapeutic recreation practice. Therapeutic Recreation Journal, 20(4), 15-30.

4. Sylvester, C.D. (1989). Impressions of the intellectual past and future of therapeutic recreation: Implications for professionalism. In D.M. Compton (Ed.), Issues in Therapeutic Recreation: A Profession in Transition (pp. 1-20). Illinois: Sagamore.

5. Ellis, G.D. (1989). The role of science in therapeutic recreation. In D.M. Comtpon (Ed.), Issues in Therapeutic Recreation: A Profession in Transition (pp. 109-123). Illlinois: Sagamore.

6. Fuhrer, M.J. (1987). Overview of outcome analysis in rehabilitation. In M.J. Fuhrer (Ed.), Rehabilitation Outcomes: Analysis and Measurement (pp.1-15). Baltimore: Paul H. Brookes.

Appendix A

LEISURE AWARENESS

Client's knowledge and understanding of leisure.

NO HELPER

7. **COMPLETE INDEPENDENCE:** Client is able to identify personal benefits of leisure involvement. Client is able to identify own leisure strengths and weaknesses. Client has realistic expectations and is able to set goals regarding leisure involvement (based on lifestyle, family situation, financial status, etc.). Client is able to identify 5 or more activities across 2 categories.

6. **MODIFIED INDEPENDENCE:** Client is able to identify personal benefits of leisure involvement. Client is able to identify own leisure strengths and weaknesses. Client has realistic expectations and is able to set goals regarding leisure involvement. Client is able to identify 3 to 4 activities across 2 categories.

HELPER

5. **MODIFIED DEPENDENCE:** Client requires cueing to identify personal benefits of leisure involvement. Client requires cueing to identify own leisure strengths and weaknesses. Client has realistic expectations and is able to set goals regarding leisure involvement. Client is able to identify 3 to 4 activities.

4. **MODIFIED DEPENDENCE WITH MINIMAL ASSISTANCE:** Client requires assistance to identify benefits of leisure involvement. Client requires assistance to identify own leisure strengths and weaknesses. Once identified, client is able to set realistic goals. Client is able to identify 1 to 2 activities.

3. **MODIFIED DEPENDENCE WITH MODERATE ASSISTANCE:** Client requires assistance to identify benefits of leisure involvement. Client has unrealistic expectations regarding leisure involvement. Client requires assistance setting realistic goals. Client is able to identify 1 to 2 activities.

2. **MODIFIED DEPENDENCE WITH MAXIMAL ASSISTANCE:** Client requires assistance to identify benefits of leisure involvement. Client has unrealistic expectations regarding leisure involvement. Client is unable to set realistic goals. Client is able to identify 1 or 2 activities.

1. **TOTAL DEPENDENCE WITH TOTAL ASSISTANCE:** Client is unable to identify benefits of leisure involvement. Client is unable to identify any activities.

LEISURE ATTITUDE

Behaviours exhibited and/or feelings demonstrated by the client which suggest attitude toward leisure involvement.

NO HELPER

7. **COMPLETE INDEPENDENCE:** Client takes initiative for own leisure involvement. Client displays a willingness to develop new leisure interest/skills. Client demonstrates feelings of enjoyment and/or satisfaction regarding leisure involvement and participation.

6. **MODIFIED INDEPENDENCE:** Client takes initiative for own leisure involvement once a program schedule has been provided. Client displays a willingness to develop new leisure interests/skill. Client demonstrates feelings of enjoyment and/or satisfaction regarding leisure involvement and participation.

HELPER

5. **MODIFIED DEPENDENCE:** Client requires cueing to initiate leisure involvement and periodic encouragement to maintain involvement. Client demonstrates discomfort with developing new leisure interests/skills. Client may or may not demonstrate feelings of enjoyment and/or satisfaction regarding leisure involvement and participation.

4. **MODIFIED DEPENDENCE WITH MINIMAL ASSISTANCE:** Client requires coaxing to initiate leisure involvement. Client requires assistance to maintain leisure involvement. Participation occurs in familiar activities only.

3. **MODIFIED DEPENDENCE WITH MODERATE ASSISTANCE:** Client requires coaxing to participate in leisure activities. Participation occurs in familiar activities only. Sporadic redirection is required to maintain client's leisure involvement.

2. **MODIFIED DEPENDENCE WITH MAXIMAL ASSISTANCE:** Client requires constant redirection to maintain leisure involvement. Client demonstrates negative feelings regarding leisure involvement and/or refuses to participate in leisure activities.

1. **TOTAL DEPENDENCE WITH TOTAL ASSISTANCE:** Due to cognitive and/or physical deficits client is unable to maintain leisure involvement.

LEISURE SKILLS

Skills possessed by the client which affect leisure involvement. Ability to independently utilize assistive devices is not considered a form of dependency.

NO HELPER

7. **COMPLETE INDEPENDENCE:** Client is able to make leisure choices based on personal interests. Client possesses the skills necessary to participate in chosen leisure activities. Client possesses the ability to independently locate and utilize leisure resources.

6. **MODIFIED INDEPENDENCE:** Client is able to make leisure choices based on personal interests. Client possesses the skills necessary to participate in chosen leisure activities. With the necessary resource material (brochures, program calendars, adaptive aids, etc.) client possesses the ability to independently locate and utilize leisure resources.

HELPER

5. **MODIFIED DEPENDENCE:** Client is able to make leisure choices based on personal interests. Client possesses the skills necessary to participate in chosen leisure activities, but requires reassurance regarding his/her competence. With cueing client possesses the ability to locate and utilize leisure resources.

4. **MODIFIED DEPENDENCE WITH MINIMAL ASSISTANCE:** Client requires assistance to make leisure choices. Client requires reassurance to participate in leisure activities. Client requires direct assistance to locate and utilize leisure resources.

3. **MODIFIED DEPENDENCE WITH MODERATE ASSISTANCE:** Client requires assistance to make leisure choices based on personal interests. Client may require skill development to participate in chosen leisure activities. Client requires direct assistance to locate and/or utilize leisure resources.

2. **MODIFIED DEPENDENCE WITH MAXIMAL ASSISTANCE:** Client is unable to make leisure choices. Selection of activities must be made for the client. Client requires skill development to participate in leisure activities. Client is unable to locate and utilize leisure resources.

1. **TOTAL DEPENDENCE WITH TOTAL ASSISTANCE:** Due to cognitive and/or physical deficits client is unable to learn age appropriate leisure skills.

CULTURAL/SOCIAL BEHAVIOURS

Specific cultural/social behaviours exhibited by the client which affect his/her ability to function effectively in leisure activities.

NO HELPER

7. **COMPLETE INDEPENDENCE:** Client displays socially acceptable manners, personal hygiene and dress. Client is courteous and tolerant of others. Client is self-directed in these areas.

6. **MODIFIED INDEPENDENCE:** Client displays socially acceptable manners, hygiene and dress, but occasionally displays poor judgement in these areas. Client is courteous and tolerant of others.

HELPER

5. **MODIFIED DEPENDENCE:** Client requires cueing regarding manners, personal hygiene, appropriate dress and/or tolerance of others. Client questions need for improvement in these areas.

4. **MODIFIED DEPENDENCE WITH MINIMAL ASSISTANCE:** Client requires assistance regarding manners, personal hygiene and/or dress. Client is tolerant of others but may become agitated.

3. **MODIFIED DEPENDENCE WITH MODERATE ASSISTANCE:** Client requires assistance regarding manners, personal hygiene and/or dress. Client may have a low tolerance of others and becomes agitated. Client may become verbally abusive and/or display a threatening manner.

2. **MODIFIED DEPENDENCE WITH MAXIMAL ASSISTANCE:** Client requires assistance regarding manners, personal hygiene and/or dress. Client has a low tolerance of others and from time to time becomes verbally and/or physically abusive. Client requires frequent intervention. Client may be resistant to intervention.

1. **TOTAL DEPENDENCE WITH TOTAL ASSISTANCE:** Client requires assistance regarding manners, personal hygiene and/or dress. Client is intolerant of others. Client is frequently verbally and/or physically abusive. Client is resistant to intervention.

INTERPERSONAL SKILLS

Client's ability to participate within various types of individual and/or group situations.

NO HELPER

7. **COMPLETE INDEPENDENCE:** Client is able to participate independently within various types of individual and/or group situations.

6. **MODIFIED INDEPENDENCE:** Client respects the needs and rights of others within the group. Client begins to trust members of the group to meet his/her esteem needs and the client, in return begins to meet the esteem needs of others by recognizing their accomplishments, but this is happening to a limited degree.

HELPER

5. **MODIFIED DEPENDENCE:** Client is able to participate in a short term task with others, the duration of the relationship being determined by the task. Client is able to do some sharing, co-operating and/or competing. The task is the focus of the group with minimal interaction between group members outside of the task.

4. **MODIFIED DEPENDENCE WITH MINIMAL ASSISTANCE:** Client is able to participate in an individual task in the presence of others. The group is more an aggregate of individuals than a group in the strict sense of the word.

3. **MODIFIED DEPENDENCE WITH MODERATE ASSISTANCE:** Client is able to participate on a one to one basis with several different individuals. Interaction is between the client and one other individual at a time.

2. **MODIFIED DEPENDENCE WITH MAXIMAL ASSISTANCE:** Client will participate on a one to one level with the primary therapist or a family member.

1. **TOTAL DEPENDENCE WITH TOTAL ASSISTANCE:** Client withdraws, isolates him/herself from others.

Adapted from Anne Mosey, Three Frames of Reference for Mental Health, p. 202.

COMMUNITY INTEGRATION SKILLS

Application of antecedent skills for successful involvement in community leisure activities.

NO HELPER

7. **COMPLETE INDEPENDENCE:** Client initiates, plans and follows through with chosen community-based leisure activities.

6. **MODIFIED INDEPENDENCE:** With the provision of the necessary resources, client initiates, plans and follows through with chosen community-based leisure activities.

HELPER

5. **MODIFIED DEPENDENCE:** With cueing and/or reassurance, client initiates, plans and follows through with chosen community-based leisure activities.

4. **MODIFIED DEPENDENCE WITH MINIMAL ASSISTANCE:** Client initiates and plans chosen community-based leisure activities. Client requires assistance with follow through.

3. **MODIFIED DEPENDENCE WITH MODERATE ASSISTANCE:** Client initiates choosing community-based leisure activities. Client requires assistance planning and following through with chosen community-based leisure activities.

2. **MODIFIED DEPENDENCE WITH MAXIMAL ASSISTANCE:** Client requires assistance initiating, planning and following through with community-based leisure activities. Even with assistance, involvement in community-based leisure activities may meet with limited success.

1. **TOTAL DEPENDENCE WITH TOTAL ASSISTANCE:** Due to cognitive and/or physical deficits client is unable to initiate, plan or follow through with community-based leisure activities.

SOCIAL CONTACT

Type and duration of social contact the client has with others.

NO HELPER

7. **COMPLETE INDEPENDENCE:** Client has a mixture of in-home/community, and family/friend social contact. Client initiates social contact. Client interacts appropriately with both family/friends and others. Social contacts are of both long (>30 minutes) and short (30 minutes or less) duration.

6. **MODIFIED INDEPENDENCE:** Client has a mixture of in-home/community, and family/friend social contact. Client initiates social contact with family/friends, and interacts appropriately with same. Client does not initiate social contact with others, but interacts appropriately in response to others. Social contacts are of both long and short duration.

HELPER

5. **MODIFIED DEPENDENCE:** Client's social contacts occur primarily in the home. Client requires cueing to initiate social contact with others. Client interacts appropriately with family/friends, but avoids social contact with others. Social contacts are of both long and short duration.

4. **MODIFIED DEPENDENCE WITH MINIMAL ASSISTANCE:** Social contact occurs primarily in the home. Client requires assistance to initiate social contact with others. Social contact consists primarily of short phrases.

3. **MODIFIED DEPENDENCE WITH MODERATE ASSISTANCE:** Social contact occurs only in the home. Social contact must be initiated by family and/or friends. Social contact consists of short, 1 or 2 word answers.

2. **MODIFIED DEPENDENCE WITH MAXIMAL ASSISTANCE:** Client does not initiate social contact. Contact by family or friends is of a custodial rather that a social nature. Client may be unable to carry on a meaningful communication.

1. **TOTAL DEPENDENCE WITH TOTAL ASSISTANCE:** No meaningful social contact.

COMMUNITY PARTICIPATION

Client's overall leisure participation pattern within their community.

NO HELPER

7. **COMPLETE INDEPENDENCE:** Client leaves their home on a regular basis and participates in a variety of leisure activities. Client demonstrates a balance of in-home and community leisure pursuits. Leisure activities are both active and passive in nature.

6. **MODIFIED INDEPENDENCE:** Client leaves their home occasionally to participate in select community leisure activities. In-home and community leisure activities are both active and passive in nature.

HELPER

5. **MODIFIED DEPENDENCE:** With encouragement and support client occasionally participates in community leisure activities. In-home and community leisure activities are both active and passive in nature.

4. **MODIFIED DEPENDENCE WITH MINIMAL ASSISTANCE:** Client participates in specialized community programs. Client may require assistance with participation. Client leaves the home to do routine activities such as taking walks, shopping, going to church, and visiting family and/or friends. Leisure activities are both active and passive in nature.

3. **MODIFIED DEPENDENCE WITH MODERATE ASSISTANCE:** Client participates in specialized community day programs. Client requires assistance to participate in community programs. Client may utilize home support leisure services. Client engages in leisure activities within the home. Leisure activities are both active and passive in nature.

2. **MODIFIED DEPENDENCE WITH MAXIMAL ASSISTANCE:** Client does not leave the home on a regular basis and does not participate in community activities. Client participates in passive leisure activities within the home.

1. **TOTAL DEPENDENCE WITH TOTAL ASSISTANCE:** Client does not participate in community or in-home leisure activities.

LEISURE COMPETENCE MEASURE©
DATA SHEET

FUNCTIONAL INDICATORS	ADM __/__/__ dd mth yr				D/C __/__/__ dd mth yr	F/U __/__/__ dd mth yr
LEISURE AWARENESS						
LEISURE ATTITUDE						
LEISURE SKILLS						
CULTURAL/SOCIAL BEHAVIOURS						
INTERPERSONAL SKILLS						
COMMUNITY INTEGRATION SKILLS						
SOCIAL CONTACT						
COMMUNITY PARTICIPATION						
TOTAL LCM SCORE (out of 56) - ADMISSION	/ 56	DISCHARGE/FOLLOW-UP			/ 56	/ 56

ADM = ADMISSION/BASELINE D/C = DISCHARGE F/U = FOLLOW-UP (≥ 2 MONTHS)

Note: Enter a value for each Functional Indicator
Enter "0" for "not assessed"

LEVELS		
	7. Complete Independence 6. Modified Independence	NO HELPER
	5. Modified Dependence 4. Modified Dependence with Minimal Assistance 3. Modified Dependence with Moderate Assistance 2. Modified Dependence with Maximal Assistance 1. Total Dependence with Total Assistance	HELPER

Appendix B

The following pages provide our rationale for scoring Cases 3 to 6, provided for practice earlier in the manual. The LCM has been scored and support material provided.

Case Study 3

Norma is a 77 year old widow living in her own home near downtown Beamsville. She lives within walking distance of the library, Senior's Centre, downtown shops and her long time friend Mabel.

Norma is in good physical health, but since her husband died one and a half years ago, she has withdrawn more and more. She used to be an active member of the Senior's Centre, going at least 3 times per week, but she has now stopped attending altogether. Even her daily walks to visit her friend Mabel have all but stopped. Norma, a once sociable, active lady, rarely leaves her home anymore. She seems content to stay at home engaging in familiar activities such as knitting, needlepoint, crossword puzzles, gardening and watching television. About once a month, Norma's daughter visits to encourage and assist Norma to put together a list of activity supplies she might need. Occasionally Norma can be persuaded by her daughter to go out to a movie. On these occasions Norma will sometimes need reminders to change her clothing and do her hair. When asked about her withdrawal from social and community activities, Norma states she finds comfort and satisfaction in staying at home and doing the things she enjoys. She says that is all she wants at this point in her life.

In the past 6 months Norma's contact with her friends has almost stopped completely. Except for visits by her daughter, there are no visitors. Norma does, however, still phone her friend Mabel once a week to talk about old times.

FUNCTIONAL INDICATORS	ADM				D/C	F/U
LEISURE AWARENESS	0					
LEISURE ATTITUDE	4					
LEISURE SKILLS	4					
CULTURAL/SOCIAL BEHAVIOURS	6					
INTERPERSONAL SKILLS	0					
COMMUNITY INTEGRATION SKILLS	2					
SOCIAL CONTACT	5					
COMMUNITY PARTICIPATION	2					
TOTAL LCM SCORE (out of 56) -ADMISSION	/ 56	DISCHARGE/FOLLOW-UP			/ 56	/ 56

ADM = ADMISSION/BASELINE D/C = DISCHARGE F/U = FOLLOW-UP (≥ 2 MONTHS)

Note: Enter a value for each Functional Indicator
Enter "0" for "not assessed"

LEVELS		
L E V E L S	7. Complete Independence 6. Modified Independence	NO HELPER
	5. Modified Dependence 4. Modified Dependence with Minimal Assistance 3. Modified Dependence with Moderate Assistance 2. Modified Dependence with Maximal Assistance 1. Total Dependence with Total Assistance	HELPER

Rationale

LEISURE AWARENESS:	Not enough information to assign a rating. Client's knowledge and understanding of leisure would have to be assessed.
LEISURE ATTITUDE:	Norma requires coaxing from her daughter to go out. Without her daughter's persuasion and presence it is very unlikely , based on the information provided, that Norma would go out herself. Also, she engages only in activities that are familiar to her (e.g., knitting, needlepoint, crossword puzzles, watching television, etc.)
LEISURE SKILLS:	Norma's daughter encourages, and physically assists Norma, to put together a list of supplies that she can then pick up for her. Without her daughter's assistance, it is very unlikely that Norma would go out to pick up her activity supplies herself.
CULTURAL/SOCIAL BEHAVIOURS:	Norma requires occasional reminders to change her clothes and do her hair.
INTERPERSONAL SKILLS:	Not enough information to assign a rating. Client's ability to participate in group situations would have to be assessed.
COMMUNITY INTEGRATION SKILLS:	Norma has very little, if any community involvement. Her daughter persuades, plans and take her to an occasional movie. Norma's daughter also goes out to pick up her activity supplies for her.
SOCIAL CONTACT:	In-home social contact only. Norma's daughter visits. Norma telephones her friend Mabel regularly.
COMMUNITY PARTICIPATION:	Norma does not leave her home on a regular basis. Involved primarily in passive, in-home activities.

Case Study 4

John, an 80 year old male, has been living in a residential home for the past 4 years. He is in reasonably good health and is able to get around on his own. John attends a day program at the local psychiatric hospital 4 days per week. Although he has been involved in regular community-based activities occasionally, John has a history of decompensating without the structure and support provided by the hospital. His interests are walking, bowling, playing cards, attending plays and listening to music. When asked, John is able to identify personal benefits of leisure, but requires some prompting. He is realistic about his leisure abilities and is able to plan realistically. John is quite willing to try new activities, but knows what he likes and does not like and will verbalize same. John often states that he enjoys his leisure involvement, but requires a gentle prompt or reminder to ensure participation. John has demonstrated an ability to make arrangements for his own leisure involvement if information is provided for him. He does, however, frequently forget the specifics about an activity, such as time and place. As a result, his ability to follow through on his plans is compromised.

John is fairly sociable and likes to take advantage of community recreation opportunities. He seems comfortable in the presence of people he does not know and will converse with them if approached. John will usually only initiate conversations with people he knows. He requires reminders with regard to hygiene and dress but will follow up on his own without further intervention. John is tolerant of group settings for short periods and is able to engage in task-oriented groups. However, his conversations and interactions with others in the group are limited.

FUNCTIONAL INDICATORS	ADM				D/C	F/U
LEISURE AWARENESS	5					
LEISURE ATTITUDE	6					
LEISURE SKILLS	5					
CULTURAL/SOCIAL BEHAVIOURS	6					
INTERPERSONAL SKILLS	5					
COMMUNITY INTEGRATION SKILLS	4					
SOCIAL CONTACT	6					
COMMUNITY PARTICIPATION	3					
TOTAL LCM SCORE (out of 56) -ADMISSION	/ 56	DISCHARGE/FOLLOW-UP			/ 56	/ 56

ADM = ADMISSION/BASELINE D/C = DISCHARGE F/U = FOLLOW-UP ($\geq$ 2 MONTHS)

Note: Enter a value for each Functional Indicator
Enter "0" for "not assessed"

LEVELS		
	7. Complete Independence 6. Modified Independence	NO HELPER
	5. Modified Dependence 4. Modified Dependence with Minimal Assistance 3. Modified Dependence with Moderate Assistance 2. Modified Dependence with Maximal Assistance 1. Total Dependence with Total Assistance	HELPER

Rationale

LEISURE AWARENESS:	John requires prompting to identify personal benefits of leisure involvement but is realistic about his abilities. He has a variety of interests across a number of activity categories (e.g., physical, music, theatre, etc.) While John meets all the requirements of level 6, he must be rated at the lower level (5) until he achieves the ability to do this without cueing.
LEISURE ATTITUDE:	John is willing to try new activities. He knows what he likes and doesn't like and can choose activities to become involved in once program information is provided to him.
LEISURE SKILLS:	John is able to choose activities that are personally meaningful and satisfying to him and also has the skills necessary to take part in these activities. However, he requires cueing (i.e., time and place of activities) to take part in those opportunities available to him.
CULTURAL/SOCIAL BEHAVIOURS:	John requires reminders regarding his hygiene and dress, but once reminded will follow through without further assistance.
INTERPERSONAL SKILLS:	John plays cards with others. This requires social interaction in a group setting. He must therefore be scored a 5. In level 4 a client participates in an individual task in the *presence* of others.
COMMUNITY INTEGRATION SKILLS:	John is able to initiate and plan his involvement in activities that are of interest to him, however, requires the structure and support provided by the day program to follow-through.
SOCIAL CONTACT:	John is comfortable in the presence of others and will talk with others if he is approached. However he will usually only initiate conversation with those people he knows.
COMMUNITY PARTICIPATION:	John attends a specialized psychiatric day program and has a history of decompensating without the structure of this program.

Case Study 5

Paul is a 35 year old male who experienced an infection causing a severe brain injury. He has right hemiplegia and requires assistance to travel in his wheelchair more than 50 feet. Paul is aphasic but with the assistance of his therapist or family members can make his needs known. He has short-term memory deficits but is able to remember events and people that are significant to him. Paul requires ongoing help with his personal needs, as well activities of daily living such as bathing and dressing. Paul does not initiate thoughts, actions or ideas in therapy or in social situations. He has not been able to identify any activities that are personally meaningful or enjoyable for him and participates for short periods only in facility programs. Paul has a short attention span and requires constant attention from his therapist to maintain involvement. Paul becomes easily agitated in group situations but is able to interact with his therapist and his brother. Paul has no visitors, other than his brother who visits approximately 3 times weekly, for anywhere from 10-30 minutes. Paul requires assistance to plan activities. Paul is not involved in any community activities, takes part in very few facility programs, and then only if his therapist takes him; he does however take part in regularly scheduled therapy sessions.

FUNCTIONAL INDICATORS	ADM				D/C	F/U
LEISURE AWARENESS	1					
LEISURE ATTITUDE	2					
LEISURE SKILLS	2					
CULTURAL/SOCIAL BEHAVIOURS	3					
INTERPERSONAL SKILLS	2					
COMMUNITY INTEGRATION SKILLS	1					
SOCIAL CONTACT	3					
COMMUNITY PARTICIPATION	2					
TOTAL LCM SCORE (out of 56) -ADMISSION	/ 56	DISCHARGE/FOLLOW-UP			/ 56	/ 56

ADM = ADMISSION/BASELINE D/C = DISCHARGE F/U = FOLLOW-UP ($\geq$ 2 MONTHS)

Note: Enter a value for each Functional Indicator
Enter "0" for "not assessed"

LEVELS		
L E V E L S	7. Complete Independence 6. Modified Independence	NO HELPER
	5. Modified Dependence 4. Modified Dependence with Minimal Assistance 3. Modified Dependence with Moderate Assistance 2. Modified Dependence with Maximal Assistance 1. Total Dependence with Total Assistance	HELPER

Rationale

LEISURE AWARENESS:	Paul is unable to identify activities that are personally meaningful or enjoyable.
LEISURE ATTITUDE:	Paul requires the constant attention of his therapist in order to participate and maintain his involvement in facility recreation programs.
LEISURE SKILLS:	Paul is unable to choose recreation activities within which to participate and relies on his therapist to take him to programs suited to his abilities. Without the direct involvement of his therapist, Paul would not take part in any programs.
CULTURAL/SOCIAL BEHAVIOURS:	Paul becomes agitated in group settings. He requires ongoing help with his personal needs, including dressing.
INTERPERSONAL SKILLS:	Paul interacts on an individual basis with his therapist and his brother. He does not interact in group settings.
COMMUNITY INTEGRATION SKILLS:	Paul is unable to initiate, plan and follow through with facility or community-based programs due to his cognitive impairment.
SOCIAL CONTACT:	Paul has no social contact other than with his brother or therapist. His interaction usually consists of short answers to questions initiated by others. He does not initiate thoughts, actions or ideas in therapy or social settings.
COMMUNITY PARTICIPATION:	Paul does participate with the direct involvement of his therapist, however, only in very few programs.

Case Study 6

Brad is a 32 year old, self-employed farmer. He was admitted to the local psychiatric hospital with severe depression. Prior to his admission, Brad's interest in his appearance and hygiene began to deteriorate. He now requires encouragement to shower and put on clean clothing. Occasionally it has been necessary to physically take him for his shower.

When interviewed by the therapeutic recreation practitioner, Brad had difficulty identifying his leisure interests. With prompting he was able to select softball, swimming, pool and euchre as activities that interested him. Brad's general knowledge of leisure activities seemed restricted to sports and games. His family revealed that Brad worked long hours on the farm and required persuasion to take time out for himself. Occasionally he played softball, went swimming and played pool. During his stay in the hospital, Brad's involvement in recreation programs has been irregular. He tends to keep to himself and only joins in after much coaxing. Brad requires staff intervention to get started in a program and ongoing supervision and encouragement to continue participating. He usually only stays for half of the program. At times, he refuses to participate even with staff encouragement. At present his primary interest is watching television, listening to music and shooting the occasional game of pool. Brad is resistive to therapeutic recreation intervention. Although leisure education and skill development are indicated, Brad states he is not interested. Other than his family, Brad has no visitors. Family members visit approximately 3-5 times per week for approximately 1-2 hours at a time.

FUNCTIONAL INDICATORS	ADM				D/C	F/U
LEISURE AWARENESS	5					
LEISURE ATTITUDE	3					
LEISURE SKILLS	4					
CULTURAL/SOCIAL BEHAVIOURS	4					
INTERPERSONAL SKILLS	0					
COMMUNITY INTEGRATION SKILLS	0					
SOCIAL CONTACT	5					
COMMUNITY PARTICIPATION	2					
TOTAL LCM SCORE (out of 56) -ADMISSION	/ 56	DISCHARGE/FOLLOW-UP			/ 56	/ 56

ADM = ADMISSION/BASELINE D/C = DISCHARGE F/U = FOLLOW-UP (≥ 2 MONTHS)

Note: Enter a value for each Functional Indicator
Enter "0" for "not assessed"

LEVELS		
	7. Complete Independence 6. Modified Independence	NO HELPER
	5. Modified Dependence 4. Modified Dependence with Minimal Assistance 3. Modified Dependence with Moderate Assistance 2. Modified Dependence with Maximal Assistance 1. Total Dependence with Total Assistance	HELPER

Rationale

LEISURE AWARENESS:	With prompting, Brad is able to identify 3-4 of his interests.
LEISURE ATTITUDE:	Brad requires coaxing and staff intervention to participate in programs; he requires ongoing supervision and encouragement to maintain his involvement; usually only stays for half the program. Take part only in those activities that are familiar to him.
LEISURE SKILLS:	Brad requires staff assistance and encouragement to choose programs that are of interest to him. Brad requires staff assistance to participate in these programs.
CULTURAL/SOCIAL BEHAVIOURS:	Brad requires reminders and encouragement in regard to his hygiene and dress. Occasionally direct staff intervention is required to take him for his shower.
INTERPERSONAL SKILLS:	Not enough information to assign a rating. Client's ability to participate in group situations would have to be assessed.
COMMUNITY INTEGRATION SKILLS:	Not enough information to assign a rating to this area. Assessment of this area is required.
SOCIAL CONTACT:	Brad socializes primarily with his family, for periods greater than 30 minutes. The visits take place in the hospital.
COMMUNITY PARTICIPATION:	Brad does not participate in community activities, occasionally takes part in facility programs with much encouragement and assistance by staff, and usually spends most of his time watching television or listening to music. Occasionally, however, he does shoot a game of pool.

Appendix C

Case Study 1

Barry has been hospitalized in a rehabilitation facility since his car accident almost a year ago. The accident left him a paraplegic. Barry is awaiting placement in an apartment of his own. In the meantime, until an apartment becomes available, he has been relocated to a rehabilitation facility near his home town.

Prior to the accident Barry was very active in sports, his primary form of leisure. Despite his initial reluctance, Barry became involved in wheelchair basketball and subsequently joined a community basketball league. He found that the feelings he is experiencing now are similar to those he felt when he played sports before his accident. Barry has arranged weekly transportation to take him to the local high-school for his league games. Barry has also developed interests and skills in art, playing the guitar, billiards and has become a member of the local sports association for the disabled. Barry is actively involved in many of the activities at the rehabilitation facility. He is usually the first to arrive and the last to leave. Barry has talked with his therapist about how much these leisure pursuits have been a positive influence in his life and how they have provided him with new challenges. Barry always appears to be pleasant and very much cares about his appearance. He is an outgoing young man who makes friends easily. Barry has many friends who visit, and whom he visits in return. His family is also very supportive, visits often and arranges for Barry to come home for visits on a regular basis.

FUNCTIONAL INDICATORS	ADM __/__/__ dd mth yr	__/__/__ dd mth yr	__/__/__ dd mth yr	__/__/__ dd mth yr	D/C __/__/__ dd mth yr	F/U __/__/__ dd mth yr
LEISURE AWARENESS						
LEISURE ATTITUDE						
LEISURE SKILLS						
CULTURAL/SOCIAL BEHAVIOURS						
INTERPERSONAL SKILLS						
COMMUNITY INTEGRATION SKILLS						
SOCIAL CONTACT						
COMMUNITY PARTICIPATION						
TOTAL LCM SCORE (out of 56) -ADMISSION	/ 56	DISCHARGE/FOLLOW-UP			/ 56	/ 56

ADM = ADMISSION/BASELINE D/C = DISCHARGE F/U = FOLLOW-UP (≥ 2 MONTHS)

Note: Enter a value for each Functional Indicator
Enter "0" for "not assessed"

Case Study 2

Anthony is a 37 year old male who sustained a severe brain injury in a motorcycle race. Prior to his accident he held an international ranking and devoted much of his time to racing. He worked occasionally as a plumber to supplement his income. Shortly after his accident his girlfriend terminated their relationship.

Anthony now requires medication to control his excitability and is somewhat rigid in his thinking. He experiences pain in his lower back which causes agitation. In the past, much of Anthony's time was spend socializing and drinking after motorcycle races. The only activities of interest to him at present are motorcycle racing and watching television. He has unrealistic expectations about being able to race again and is unable to identify why it might be important for him to be involved in other activities. Anthony requires assistance to participate in facility programs and often if in a program, requires constant re-direction by his therapist to maintain his involvement. He does not self-initiate, often lacks the ability to focus, his judgement is impaired and at times he is at risk for his own safety. While Anthony does not participate for long in group settings, he does interact on an individual level with his therapist and with family members. He interacts reasonably well with those he knows; his interaction with others is often inappropriate in that he talks excessively, tends to confabulate and is socially disinhibited. In group situations Anthony is often intolerant of others and at times has become verbally and physically aggressive. Anthony requires physical intervention in regard to his manners and to dress appropriately for the weather; he often resists the assistance provided by his therapist. He requires assistance from his therapist to plan and follow through on outings to the community, and often these outings have to be cut short due to Anthony's fatigue and/or behaviour. Anthony, at this point, does not participate in community programs, spends most of his time watching television in his room, and only takes part in facility programs with direct assistance from his therapist.

FUNCTIONAL INDICATORS	ADM __/__/__ dd mth yr	__/__/__ dd mth yr	__/__/__ dd mth yr	__/__/__ dd mth yr	D/C __/__/__ dd mth yr	F/U __/__/__ dd mth yr
LEISURE AWARENESS						
LEISURE ATTITUDE						
LEISURE SKILLS						
CULTURAL/SOCIAL BEHAVIOURS						
INTERPERSONAL SKILLS						
COMMUNITY INTEGRATION SKILLS						
SOCIAL CONTACT						
COMMUNITY PARTICIPATION						
TOTAL LCM SCORE (out of 56) -ADMISSION	/ 56	DISCHARGE/FOLLOW-UP			/ 56	/ 56

ADM = ADMISSION/BASELINE D/C = DISCHARGE F/U = FOLLOW-UP (≥ 2 MONTHS)

<u>Note</u>: Enter a value for each Functional Indicator
Enter "0" for "not assessed"

Case Study 3

Norma is a 77 year old widow living in her own home near downtown Beamsville. She lives within walking distance of the library, Senior's Centre, downtown shops and her long time friend Mabel.

Norma is in good physical health, but since her husband died one and a half years ago, she has withdrawn more and more. She used to be an active member of the Senior's Centre, going at least 3 times per week, but she has now stopped attending altogether. Even her daily walks to visit her friend Mabel have all but stopped. Norma, a once sociable, active lady, rarely leaves her home anymore. She seems content to stay at home engaging in familiar activities such as knitting, needlepoint, crossword puzzles, gardening and watching television. About once a month, Norma's daughter visits to encourage and assist Norma to put together a list of activity supplies she might need. Occasionally Norma can be persuaded by her daughter to go out to a movie. On these occasions Norma will sometimes need reminders to change her clothing and do her hair. When asked about her withdrawal from social and community activities, Norma states she finds comfort and satisfaction in staying at home and doing the things she enjoys. He says that is all she wants at this point in her life.

In the past 6 months Norma's contact with her friends has almost stopped completely. Except for visits by her daughter, there are no visitors. Norma does, however, still phone her friend Mabel once a week to talk about old times.

FUNCTIONAL INDICATORS	ADM _/_/_ dd mth yr	_/_/_ dd mth yr	_/_/_ dd mth yr	_/_/_ dd mth yr	D/C _/_/_ dd mth yr	F/U _/_/_ dd mth yr
LEISURE AWARENESS						
LEISURE ATTITUDE						
LEISURE SKILLS						
CULTURAL/SOCIAL BEHAVIOURS						
INTERPERSONAL SKILLS						
COMMUNITY INTEGRATION SKILLS						
SOCIAL CONTACT						
COMMUNITY PARTICIPATION						
TOTAL LCM SCORE (out of 56) -ADMISSION	/ 56	**DISCHARGE/FOLLOW-UP**			/ 56	/ 56

ADM = ADMISSION/BASELINE D/C = DISCHARGE F/U = FOLLOW-UP (≥ 2 MONTHS)

Note: Enter a value for each Functional Indicator
Enter "0" for "not assessed"

Case Study 4

John, an 80 year old male, has been living in a residential home for the past 4 years. He is in reasonably good health and is able to get around on his own. John attends a day program at the local psychiatric hospital 4 days per week. Although he has been involved in regular community-based activities occasionally, John has a history of decompensating without the structure and support provided by the hospital. His interests are walking, bowling, playing cards, attending plays and listening to music. When asked, John is able to identify personal benefits of leisure, but requires some prompting. He is realistic about his leisure abilities and is able to plan realistically. John is quite willing to try new activities, but knows what he likes and does not like and will verbalize same. John often states that he enjoys his leisure involvement, but requires a gentle prompt or reminder to ensure participation. John has demonstrated an ability to make arrangements for his own leisure involvement if information is provided for him. He does, however, frequently forget the specifics about an activity, such as time and place. As a result, his ability to follow through on his plans is compromised.

John is fairly sociable and likes to take advantage of community recreation opportunities. He seems comfortable in the presence of people he does not know and will converse with them if approached. John will usually only initiate conversations with people he knows. He requires reminders with regard to hygiene and dress but will follow up on his own without further intervention. John is tolerant of group settings for short periods and is able to engage in task-oriented groups. However, his conversations and interactions with others in the group are limited.

FUNCTIONAL INDICATORS	**ADM** __/__/__ dd mth yr	__/__/__ dd mth yr	__/__/__ dd mth yr	__/__/__ dd mth yr	**D/C** __/__/__ dd mth yr	**F/U** __/__/__ dd mth yr
LEISURE AWARENESS						
LEISURE ATTITUDE						
LEISURE SKILLS						
CULTURAL/SOCIAL BEHAVIOURS						
INTERPERSONAL SKILLS						
COMMUNITY INTEGRATION SKILLS						
SOCIAL CONTACT						
COMMUNITY PARTICIPATION						
TOTAL LCM SCORE (out of 56) -ADMISSION	/ **56**	**DISCHARGE/FOLLOW-UP**			/ **56**	/ **56**

ADM = ADMISSION/BASELINE D/C = DISCHARGE F/U = FOLLOW-UP ($\geq$ 2 MONTHS)

Note: Enter a value for each Functional Indicator
Enter "0" for "not assessed"

Case Study 5

Paul is a 35 year old male who experienced an infection causing a severe brain injury. He has right hemiplegia and requires assistance to travel in his wheelchair more than 50 feet. Paul is aphasic but with the assistance of his therapist or family members can make his needs known. He has short-term memory deficits but is able to remember events and people that are significant to him. Paul requires ongoing help with his personal needs, as well activities of daily living such as bathing and dressing. Paul does not initiate thoughts, actions or ideas in therapy or in social situations. He has not been able to identify any activities that are personally meaningful or enjoyable for him and participates for short periods only in facility programs. Paul has a short attention span and requires constant attention from his therapist to maintain involvement. Paul becomes easily agitated in group situations but is able to interact with his therapist and his brother. Paul has no visitors, other than his brother who visits approximately 3 times weekly, for anywhere from 10-30 minutes. Paul requires assistance to plan activities. Paul is not involved in any community activities, takes part in very few facility programs, and then only if his therapist takes him; he does however take part in regularly scheduled therapy sessions.

FUNCTIONAL INDICATORS	ADM __/__/__ dd mth yr	__/__/__ dd mth yr	__/__/__ dd mth yr	__/__/__ dd mth yr	D/C __/__/__ dd mth yr	F/U __/__/__ dd mth yr
LEISURE AWARENESS						
LEISURE ATTITUDE						
LEISURE SKILLS						
CULTURAL/SOCIAL BEHAVIOURS						
INTERPERSONAL SKILLS						
COMMUNITY INTEGRATION SKILLS						
SOCIAL CONTACT						
COMMUNITY PARTICIPATION						
TOTAL LCM SCORE (out of 56) -ADMISSION	/ 56	DISCHARGE/FOLLOW-UP			/ 56	/ 56

ADM = ADMISSION/BASELINE D/C = DISCHARGE F/U = FOLLOW-UP (≥ 2 MONTHS)

Note: Enter a value for each Functional Indicator
Enter "0" for "not assessed"

Case Study 6

Brad is a 32 year old, self-employed farmer. He was admitted to the local psychiatric hospital with severe depression. Prior to his admission, Brad's interest in his appearance and hygiene began to deteriorate. He now requires encouragement to shower and put on clean clothing. Occasionally it has been necessary to physically take him for his shower.

When interviewed by the therapeutic recreation practitioner, Brad had difficulty identifying his leisure interests. With prompting he was able to select softball, swimming, pool and euchre as activities that interested him. Brad's general knowledge of leisure activities seemed restricted to sports and games. His family revealed that Brad worked long hours on the farm and required persuasion to take time out for himself. Occasionally he played softball, went swimming and played pool. During his stay in the hospital, Brad's involvement in recreation programs has been irregular. He tends to keep to himself and only joins in after much coaxing. Brad requires staff intervention to get started in a program and ongoing supervision and encouragement to continue participating. He usually only stays for half of the program. At times, he refuses to participate even with staff encouragement. At present his primary interest is watching television, listening to music and shooting the occasional game of pool. Brad is resistive to therapeutic recreation intervention. Although leisure education and skill development are indicated, Brad states he is not interested. Other than his family, Brad has no visitors. Family members visit approximately 3-5 times per week for approximately 1-2 hours at a time.

FUNCTIONAL INDICATORS	ADM __/__/__ dd mth yr	__/__/__ dd mth yr	__/__/__ dd mth yr	__/__/__ dd mth yr	D/C __/__/__ dd mth yr	F/U __/__/__ dd mth yr
LEISURE AWARENESS						
LEISURE ATTITUDE						
LEISURE SKILLS						
CULTURAL/SOCIAL BEHAVIOURS						
INTERPERSONAL SKILLS						
COMMUNITY INTEGRATION SKILLS						
SOCIAL CONTACT						
COMMUNITY PARTICIPATION						
TOTAL LCM SCORE (out of 56) -ADMISSION	/ 56	DISCHARGE/FOLLOW-UP			/ 56	/ 56

ADM = ADMISSION/BASELINE D/C = DISCHARGE F/U = FOLLOW-UP (≥ 2 MONTHS)

Note: Enter a value for each Functional Indicator
Enter "0" for "not assessed"

Appendix D

LCM Subscales - Glossary

realistic expectations:	outcomes that can be achieved given the strengths and weaknesses of the client, the time available to the therapeutic recreation specialist, and the resources available
5 or more activities across 2 categories:	activity categories are based on the LeisureScope (Nall-Shenk, 1983) categories used to help classify leisure activities
cueing:	verbal direction provided during the performance of a task
assistance:	physical help provided during the performance of a task. In the case of the Leisure Awareness and Leisure Attitude subscales this implies the physical presence of the therapeutic recreation specialist while he/she works closely with the client to identify goals, benefits, etc.
periodic encouragement:	intermittent encouragement falling short of specific direction
coaxing:	encouragement provided on a more intensive level but not entailing specific direction about how to complete the task
sporadic re-direction:	intermittent guidance provided to help the client re-focus on the task and keep on track
constant re-direction:	intensive guidance requiring the constant presence and attention of the therapeutic recreation specialist to keep the client on track
reassurance:	used in the Leisure Skills subscale and equivalent to periodic encouragement on the Leisure Attitude subscale (see above)
socially acceptable: (e.g., manners, hygiene, etc.)	that degree of presentation and performance that conforms with the expectations set by the cultural norms of the client's society
frequent intervention:	used in the cultural/social behaviours subscale and equivalent to constant re-direction on the Leisure Attitude subscale (see above)
interacts appropriately:	this implies a degree of interaction considered appropriate to the client's societal mores. Inappropriate behaviour can be shown by under performance (e.g., failure to interact), by inappropriate interaction (e.g., verbal aggression, swearing), or by over interaction (excessive talking)
specialized community programs:	those programs which cater to the needs of specific groups or types of of clients (e.g., the elderly)
specialized community day programs:	are similar to specialized community programs but provide a greater degree of protection and support, cater to clients with more complex disabilities and might be providing a family relief role (e.g., Alzheimer day programs)
home support leisure service:	those services which cater to the needs of clients in their home (e.g., the Home Library Service)

www.ingramcontent.com/pod-product-compliance
Lightning Source LLC
LaVergne TN
LVHW080045210926
848481LV00011B/3286